THE FOLKLORE SOCIETY
MISTLETOE SERIES

PRIMITIVE RELIGION AND HEALING

Other titles in the Mistletoe Series

The Last of the Astrologers
William Lilly
ed. K. M. Briggs

The Journey to the Other World
Ed. H. R. E. Davidson

A Collection of Highland Rites and Customes
Robert Kirk
ed. J. L. Campbell

Legends of Icelandic Magicians
Ed. Jacqueline Simpson

The Secret Common-wealth
Robert Kirk
ed. Stewart Sanderson

Ballad Studies
Ed. E. B. Lyle

Symbols of Power
Ed. H. R. E. Davidson

Ritual Animal Disguise
E. C. Cawte

Animals in Folklore
Eds. J. R. Porter and W. M. S. Russell

The Jack-in-the-Green
Roy Judge

PRIMITIVE RELIGION AND HEALING

A study of folk medicine in North-East Brazil

Paul V. A. Williams

Published by D. S. Brewer
and Rowman and Littlefield
for the Folklore Society
1979

Published by D. S. Brewer
240 Hills Road, Cambridge
and P. O. Box 9, Woodbridge, Suffolk IP12 3DF
First published in the U.S.A. 1979 by
Rowman and Littlefield, Totowa, N.J.

British Library Cataloguing in Publication Data
Williams, Paul V A
Primitive religion and healing. – (Mistletoe series).
1. Folk medicine – Brazil – Recôncauo
I. Title II. Folklore Society
III, Series
615'.882'09814 GR133.B6

ISBN 0-85991-055-5
U.S. ISBN 0-8476-6222-5

Printed and Bound in Great Britain by
REDWOOD BURN LIMITED
Trowbridge & Esher

FOR ROSIE

CONTENTS

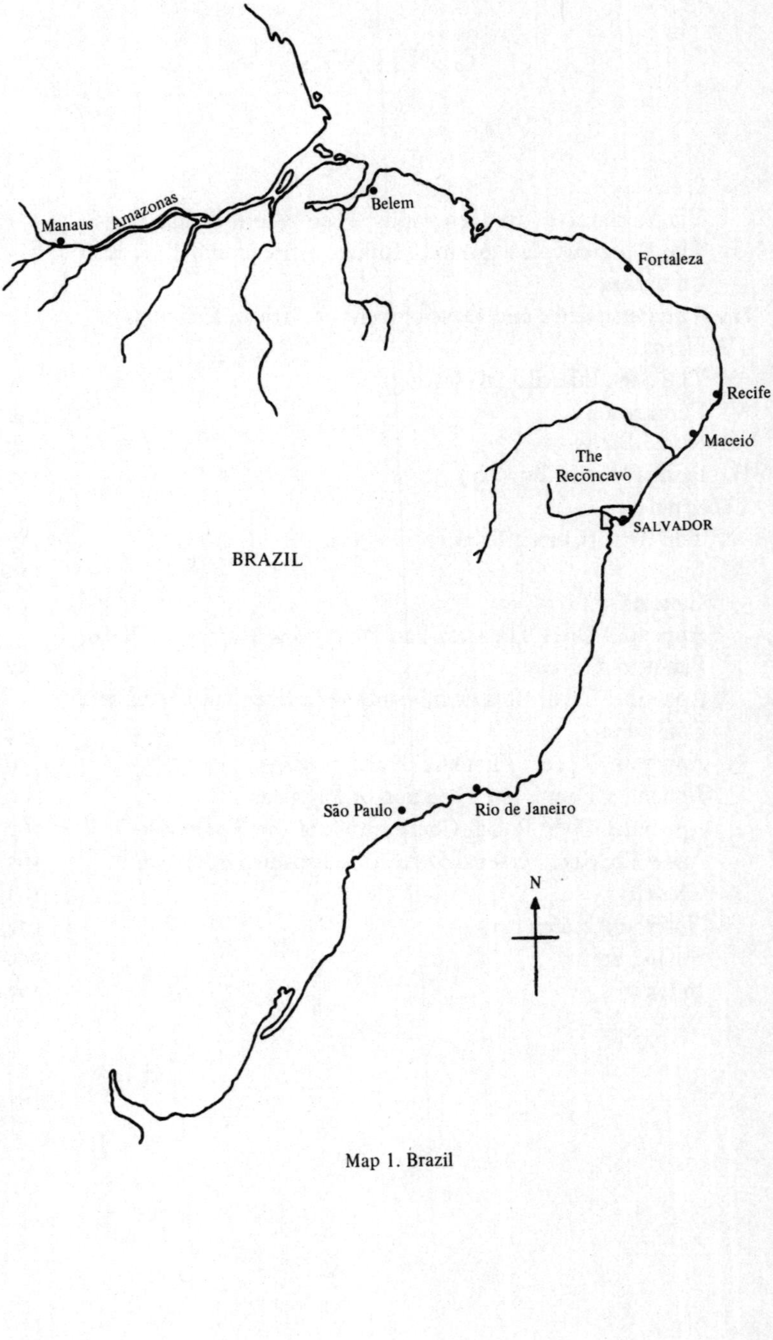
Manaus
Amazonas
Belem
Fortaleza
Recife
Maceió
The
Recôncavo
SALVADOR
BRAZIL
São Paulo
Rio de Janeiro
N

Map 1. Brazil

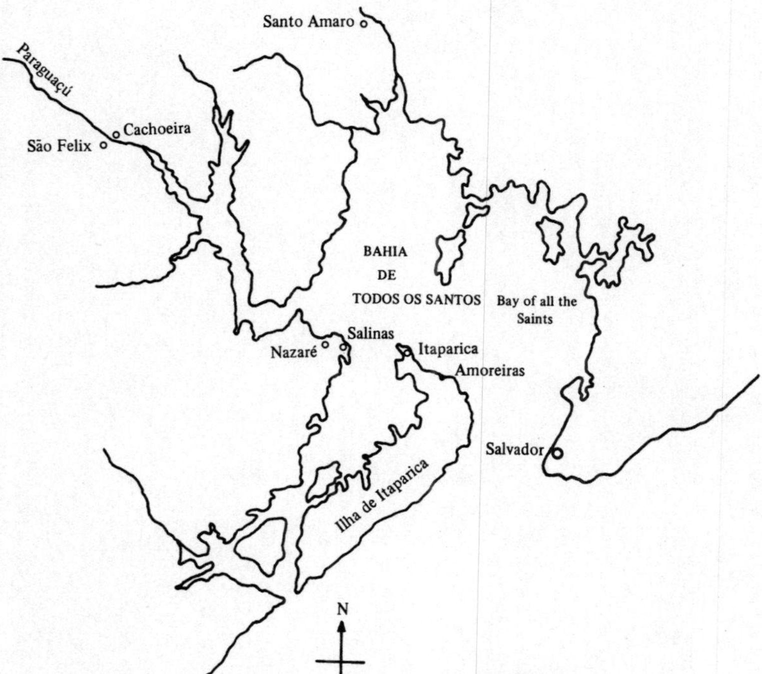

Map 2. Recôncavo

PREFACE

This book is based on findings from fieldwork carried out over a ten-month period from July 1973 to April 1974 in the Recôncavo, working from three centres: Itaparica, on the island of Itaparica in the Bay of All the Saints; Cachoeira, a town on the River Paraguaçú some eighty-five miles from Salvador; and Salvador, the state capital. From these centres regular trips were made to villages and outlying rural districts to obtain as representative a survey as possible within the defined geographical limits. Itaparica was chosen as a centre for study because of its semi-isolation from the rest of the Recôncavo as an island. It is now linked to the mainland by a regular ferry service and is joined on the south-western side by a bridge, but was for many years accessible only by canoe or similar small craft. Cachoeira, on the other hand, was chosen by virtue of its central position in the interior of the Recôncavo, having long been a key trading centre and market town providing a link between the *sertão*[1] and the coast, based on economic factors but providing a centre for cultural exchange at the same time. It has a much larger population than Itaparica, although Itaparica is the capital of the island, and has in the past been more affected by external influences, notably the German-owned tobacco factories situated at São Félix immediately opposite Cachoeira on the River Paraguaçú. Cachoeira reached its peak in terms of economic prosperity and population density in the middle of the nineteenth century and has now declined in both these respects, but continues to be a focal point in the social and economic life of the Recôncavo. Salvador, the state capital, with its population of over a million, was chosen as representative of a large urban centre in the process of industrialization and also as the nucleus of the Recôncavo. This concentrated fieldwork was complemented by a stay of two weeks in Rio de Janeiro (1973) and Galicia (1975) respectively. The period spend in Galicia enabled me to establish definitively the Iberian origin of certain practices and to trace other similarities in present-day curing practices.

In and around each of the three centres, contact was established with a number of informants involved in different ways with *curandeirismo*, and interviews were carried out with them covering as wide a field of inquiry as possible within the scope of the study, to obtain a balanced general viewpoint and, simultaneously, a corpus of data of a more specific and peculiar nature. Informants were of both sexes and all ages, but tended to belong to lower socio-economic groups.[2] Through informants, entry as an observer was obtained to a number of rituals of a normally secret or restricted nature, and in some cases the taking of photographs and/or making of tape-recordings was permitted as a favour. Regular attendance at *Candomblé* festivals and rites of a public nature, and at *sessões espíritas* (*séances*) complemented findings in personal interviews and rituals such as those mentioned above.

Informants were on the whole willing to provide assistance, though some insisted on limiting the information they were prepared to give, principally on account of an obligation not to reveal certain cult secrets they had sworn to keep on the occasion of their initiation into the priestly hierarchy, or out of fear that individual curing methods, considered by them to be particularly effective, might become known to rival *curandeiros*. Rivalry was not concealed, and there was considerable acrimony between many *curandeiros* and their respective followers within towns and villages, and this was often reflected in contradictory information being given.[3]

Informants are referred to in the text by means of an initial and number. In each case, the initial refers to the location in which the informant lived (e.g. I = Itaparica, C = Cachoeira, S = Salvador, P = Pataxó, R = Rio de Janeiro and G = Galicia) and the number to the informant in question. Basic biographical details in respect of each informant are given in Appendix Six.

All incantations and prayers that were collected in the original Portuguese have been translated as far as possible into English, and the English form only is given. This is not an ideal compromise, but to have given both English and Portuguese versions would have considerably lengthened the book and hence have contributed substantially to printing costs. The original Portuguese can be found in the thesis on which this book is based, lodged in the library of St Andrews University under the title: *Curandeirismo in the Recôncavo of Bahia: A Study in Cultural Syncretism Based on the Fusion of African, Indigenous and European Curing Practices*. With regard to transcribing passages from books and other sources written in languages other than English (particularly Portuguese and Spanish), English versions have only been given whenever this has been deemed necessary to allow for an adequate understanding of the text. Prayers and incantations have been translated literally so as to ensure accuracy; hence the English is often very stilted. I have adopted the policy of leaving most common names and most of the vocabulary concerning ritual and illness in the original Portuguese.

All African and Tupi terms are transcribed according to recognized Brazilian Portuguese orthography. Where it has been impossible to identify African terms, these have been transcribed likewise in the text for ease of reading, and phonetically in Appendix Three. Each word or group of words transcribed in such a way in the text is marked with an asterisk and is identified in Appendix Three by its relevant page number. A glossary is provided for most foreign terms employed.

I am indebted to the following people and institutions without whose help this book might never have been written: Dr Celso da Rocha Miranda, K.B.E.; Shell International Marine Ltd; the Brazilian Government; the British Academy; Dr Ramakrishna Bhagavan dos Santos; Professor Frederico Edelweiss; Dr Vivaldo da Costa Lima; Teresinha Fróes Assunção; Glória Carvalho; Peter Craddock; The Russell Trust (University of St Andrews); Dr G. S. Harris, Department of Chemistry, University of St Andrews; and Professor D. J. Gifford, also of the University of St Andrews, for all his invaluable advice and assistance.

This book is dedicated to my wife, who has given me so much help and tireless encouragement to complete the project.

P.V.A.W.

Winchester College
1978

CHAPTER I

THE RECÔNCAVO: ITS GEOGRAPHY, HISTORY AND PEOPLE

Brazil, the fifth largest country in the world (area 3,286,647 square miles),[1] is divided into twenty-five states of which Bahia is one of the largest (342,000 square miles).[2] The capital, Salvador (or Bahia, the name being applied locally both to the state and the capital), has a population of 1,314,000 (as calculated in 1974) out of a total national population of 104 million.[1] Bahia, together with the states of Sergipe, Alagoas, Paraíba, Pernambuco, Ceará and Rio Grande do Norte, falls within the larger region known as the Nordeste,[3] which was once the economically dominant area of Brazil but which has now declined in favour of the more prosperous industrial and urbanized south, balanced by the decline in importance of the traditional plantation system of agriculture which has occurred simultaneously. The Nordeste still supports 25 per cent of the total population of Brazil on only 11 per cent of her land.[4]

Bahia is still an important sugar producer, sugar cane being the major crop grown in the coastal zone from Paraíba southwards, and also produces 95 per cent of Brazil's cocoa. This industry is centred in the south of the state around Ilhéus. Coffee, sisal and piassava are grown on a lesser scale, and tobacco continues to be an important export. Natural deposits have begun to be exploited more recently, and Bahia now produces 100 per cent of Brazil's barite, 96 per cent of magnesite, 81 per cent of petroleum and 73 per cent of her lead.[5] Copper-ore deposits have been discovered, and natural gas and oil are also being exploited. The industrial centre of Aratú, on the outskirts of Salvador, is the site of an important aluminium smelting plant.

However, to a large extent, technical and industrial progress in this part of Brazil has been considerably more rapid than advances in the social services, and educational and medical facilities, particularly in rural areas, tend to be deficient. In the industrial zone of the south of Brazil, for example, 1974 statistics show that there is one doctor per 1,600 inhabitants and one hospital bed available per 200, while in the north-east, there is only one doctor per 5,700 and only one hospital bed per 630.

The Recôncavo is a fairly narrow strip of land surrounding the Bay of All the Saints (see the maps on pages vi–vii). It is about sixty miles long and about thirty miles wide at its widest point. It is an exceptionally fertile region, well-watered and with a soil type (*massapé*) particularly suited to the cultivation of sugar and tobacco. It was formerly a centre of large landholdings, owned by the type of rural aristocracy which characterized colonial Brazil, and founded on slavery and a patriarchal social system.[6] It was one of the first areas to be colonized by the Portuguese, Salvador having been established in 1502 as one of the first permanent European trading posts, primarily concerned with the export of Brazil-wood.[7] The actual discovery of Brazil in 1500 is attributed to Pedro Alvares Cabral, but recent research has shown it is likely that Phoenician traders reached the north-east coast in the sixth century B.C.[8]

In the early years of the sixteenth century, French trade in Brazil-wood predominated over Portuguese, but in 1530, to establish Portuguese supremacy, the authorities in Lisbon divided the coastal area of Brazil into twelve *capitanias*, each administered by representatives of the Crown, and colonization began to increase. Sugar was introduced from Madeira shortly after this, and the first African slaves began to be imported in 1538 to work on the sugar plantations.[9] By 1587, there were already forty-seven *engenhos* (sugar plantations and mills) within a radius of Salvador.[10]

The first Portuguese immigrants were, for the most part, *degredados*, individuals virtually expelled from Portugal for criminal, religious or political offences; or impoverished nobles, with prostitutes and orphan girls sent by the court to provide wives for the male immigrants. Many mixed with women of Indian stock from indigenous tribes who had, on the whole, proved friendly since the arrival of the first traders, with whom they had cooperated, exchanging labour and the Brazil-wood of their forests for trinkets and axes.[11]

The coastal tribes of Brazil in the early sixteenth century were, for the most part, a fairly settled and culturally advanced people in comparison with the tribes inhabiting the interior. The area around Bahia (Salvador) was settled by Tupinambá and Tupiniquin tribes, who were of a peaceful disposition in contrast to the fierce and culturally more backward Botocudo who sacked and laid waste Tupinambá and Tupiniquin villages periodically, even after colonization, killing Indians and Portuguese alike.[12]

The Indians contributed in many ways to the foundations of Brazilian culture, from methods of preparing food to the introduction of the hammock to replace the European bed, and, even more significantly, to the physical appearance and characteristics of the average Brazilian today.[13] Their contribution to the religious sphere will be discussed in the next chapter.

The significance of the early sugar-plantation economy, however, must be seen in a much wider perspective and not simply as the means whereby the Portuguese Crown and the early colonizers derived income. It laid the foundations for a whole system of land tenure and land use which persisted for centuries, and still persists in some areas.[14] In the same way, it provided a base for Brazilian social and economic institutions and is thus of enduring importance. In physical terms, it should be seen as the underlying cause of the intense miscegenation which characterizes the state of Bahia,[15] and of the consequent cultural syncretism that is a marked feature of life in Salvador and the Recôncavo.

CHAPTER II

THE RELIGIOUS BACKGROUND: INDIAN, AFRICAN AND EUROPEAN INFLUENCES

There are various religious elements underlying *curandeirismo* as it is practised today in the Recôncavo of Bahia, and these should be examined initially in their historical perspective. First, there is the Indian, who in the early years of the Portuguese Empire played an important role in setting the cultivation of sugar in motion and establishing Brazil as one of the main sources of sugar in the world. The Portuguese had soon discovered after their arrival that the type of soil along the north-east coast, in particular the type called *massapé* in the area around the bay of Salvador, was highly suited for the cultivation of sugar, and that fortunes were to be made on the European sugar markets. The first settlements were in Pernambuco, around the town of Recife, and what is known as the Recôncavo of Bahia, namely the strip of land that surrounds the Bay of All the Saints. There were many Indians of Tupi stock in this area at the time and the Portuguese found little difficulty in rounding them up and forming them into gangs. The first plantations were cut into the jungle with Indian labour,[1] but as sugar markets increased and more and more labour was required of the Indian, it became apparent that as far as extreme physical exertion was concerned, he was inadequate and unreliable. He was not naturally inclined towards prolonged physical effort of this nature because he was a nomad, used to surviving by means of the bow and arrow, collecting all the fruits that grew wild in the jungle and cultivating only the minimum quantity of manioc and maize that was essential for the survival of the tribe. The notion of monoculture was totally foreign to him, and his metabolism deteriorated as a result of the new pattern of life imposed upon him by the Portuguese. His traditional diet was no longer sufficiently sustaining during the long periods of physical labour to which he was subjected, and whole tribes became ill and died because of this and because of the introduction of European diseases to which the Indian had no immunity. It was clear that a different form of labour had to be imported from elsewhere.

The religion practised by the Indians at the time of colonization is little different from that found today among tribes of related stocks who still preserve their tribal units. Basically animistic in character, and including worship of the sun and moon, the religious beliefs and the ritual practices of the tribe centred around the figure of the *pagé*, who fulfilled the dual function of priest and medicine man, functions inseparable in many cults throughout the world. Belief was founded on myth, and the Tupi-Guarani traced their origins back to a Creation myth, which included the Flood myth found among so many other peoples.[2] They believed in a Paradise or Promised Land far to the east, the object of numerous quests and migrations under the messianic leadership of certain *pagés*.[3] A number of these traits clearly coincided with Christian belief, despite the greater sophistication of the latter, and were therefore easily assimilated in the process of conversion. Other common beliefs and practices allied indigenous religions to those of the Africans who arrived later, and the same process of absorbtion and assimilation took place.

The Jesuits, according to Freyre, 'sought to destroy, or at least to castrate, every virile expression of religion or artistic culture that was not in agreement with Catholic morality and European conventions'.[4] Moreover, they settled the Indians into communities, thus disrupting their established nomadic way of life and many of the religious traditions and practices that were an integral part of it, and usurped the authority of the *pagé*, thus disintegrating the religious life of the community at its roots. In catechizing the children, the Jesuits preserved certain songs and dances, but transformed former objects of fear, representations of spirits and demons, into comic figures, thus weakening the hold of totemism on successive generations[5] and using the indoctrinated children as a powerful tool in the conversion of their elders.

Those Indians that remained in the coastal area, therefore, and who did not disappear inland away from the colonizers and the Jesuits who accompanied them, were soon converted, or at least subjected, to Christianity in a way which permitted few of their original beliefs and practices to survive. Their positive contribution to the amalgam of beliefs underlying religious practices in the north-east today was small in comparison with African and European elements, and the apparently Indian features which are found today in *Candomblé de caboclo*, such as the inclusion of Indian saints in worship and the placating of their spirits, are later introductions on the part of *Candomblé de caboclo* adherents. These elements will be discussed more fully in the next chapter.

Metropolitan Portuguese slave-traders were already familiar with certain African peoples, especially the Yoruba, whom they had been taking as slaves since 1452.[6] They knew them to be good workers, and it was thus that the importation of slaves into Brazil began. It is difficult to establish exactly from what parts of Africa slaves came in the sixteenth and seventeenth centuries. The geographical terminology of Portuguese sailors was vague, and slaves in Brazil could often only give the name of their place of embarkation and the name of the district where they had lived, and not the name of the specific tribe to which they belonged.[7] Slaves were frequently described as being from Guiné, Costa da Mina or Angola, or even simply as *preto da Guiné* (black man from Guinea), *negro da Costa* (Negro from the Coast) or *peça da India* (specimen from India).[8] Nagô, another term used, was the name given by the French to those people who spoke Yoruba and its related dialects.[9] It subsequently became a generic term for the language which evolved as a result of the mingling of the different Yoruba and other tribes through forced co-habitation on the sugar plantations in Brazil. It became a common language among different African peoples, who used it as an instrument of communication. As their religions fused and syncretized, establishing a tradition of African ritual, so did their languages; and as their acculturation with Portuguese elements, in particular the Portuguese language, proceeded, Nagô became a secondary means of communication and began to be spoken only as a ritual language in religious observances.[10]

Guiné, to Portuguese sailors, comprised a region covering almost the whole of the West coast of Africa, from Cameroon to Angola (Ott 1955:I, 58), whereas now it is taken to designate the small area of ex-Portuguese possessions in that area. There is even evidence that slaves came from as far away as Mozambique.[11] Ott has drawn attention to another source of confusion with regard to the true ethnic origins of certain African slaves. It appears that Brazilian slave buyers would stipulate that certain batches of slaves originate from a particular tribe or country. The slave-traders, not wanting to lose the business, would then alter the nationalities of the slaves they were currently transporting in order to please the Brazilian buyers.[12]

The traffic was controlled from Portugal, and in the early sixteenth century each *senhor de engenho* (sugar-plantation owner) was allowed to import 120 slaves per *engenho* from Guiné and São Thomé.[13] Bahia was, at this time, the capital of Brazil, and also an important centre of trade, not only now for Brazil-wood, but also for sugar from the multiplying *engenhos* of the Recôncavo. During the seventeenth century, although statistics are unreliable, the Negro population increased considerably, as the extensive tables given by Pierson demonstrate (1967:129–33).

In 1763, the government moved to Rio de Janeiro, but Bahia continued to be an important centre of trade and of slave traffic. The traffic with Africa was not merely one way, for considerable exports were made from Brazil back to Africa. Tobacco was being shipped there as early as 1710, and for over a century Portuguese colonies on the west coast of Africa absorbed some 35 per cent of Bahia's production. Sugar, manioc meal, *aguardente* (brandy, i.e. sugar-cane brandy) and cowries were also exported to such an extent that there are reports of French travellers referring to Bahia as 'New Guinea', while the African natives of Guinea referred to the outer world as Bahia.[14]

The trade exchange proved so profitable that in 1795 the king of Dahomey sent two ambassadors to the Portuguese authorities in Bahia to propose a commercial treaty assuring the exclusive provision of slaves to the port of Ouidah. In the end, the proposal was rejected on the grounds that it was not prudent to import too many slaves of the same nation to one area.[15]

Of the Sudanese groups, the Gêge (from the Porto Novo area of Dahomey) were brought over in large numbers in the seventeenth century, when the Dahomean peoples were enjoying supremacy over the other peoples of the slave coast, but numbers dwindled later. The Yoruba, on the other hand, despite their long contact with the Portuguese and their early introduction into Brazil as slaves, were only brought to Brazil in large numbers in the eighteenth and nineteenth centuries, when they were suppressed by the Dahomeans, and for this reason their influence has tended to predominate over that of other peoples, especially in Bahia.

Ott, basing his research on information in the public archives of Bahia, the *Ordens Régias* and over 130 manuscripts containing contracts of sale of slaves in the municipal archives, as well as ecclesiastical registers, concludes that in the eighteenth century the majority of slaves in the capital were of Sudanese origin, in which he includes the group known as Nagô, while in the *sertão* at the same period, the majority were of Bantu origin, a good half being from Angola. This preponderance of Sudanese in the capital prevailed into the early nineteenth century according to sale contracts, while Recôncavo parish registers of the nineteenth century record almost equal proportions of Bantu and Sudanese, although there seems to have been a preponderance of Sudanese in certain larger centres of population like Nazaré.[16] The Hausa, who were the principal Moslem group, were imported on a lesser scale, but because of their more advanced cultural level, they played an important part in the development of regional culture.

More and more slaves were required continually for the Recôncavo sugar plantations, and when, in 1815, Portugal adhered to the Vienna Convention abolishing slave-trading north of the equator, Bahia continued, and even augmented, the traffic with Ouidah and Lagos, paying only lip-service to the Convention.[17]

The form that slavery took in Brazil bears marked differences from that in North America and other areas of the New World. This has been studied and commented on at length by Gilberto Freyre in *Casa Grande e Senzala* (1933) and *Sobrados e Mucambos* (1936), and his conclusions are borne out by the reports of many early travellers. Burton commented, 'nowhere, even in oriental countries, has the "bitter draught" so little of gall in it'.[18] Miscegenation was widespread, and a network of intimate personal relationships distinguished slavery in Brazil from slavery in North America.[19]

Another important feature was that, while it was considered unwise to form large groups of slaves emanating from the same tribe, distinguishable tribal units on the plantations were not deliberately split up, and this enabled the African to maintain his own beliefs, customs and racial integrity, and to transmit his culture to his children, which was not the case in English-administered territories.[20] Smaller ethnic groups tended to be absorbed by larger ones, with the exception of the influential Hausa group, which remained important in Bahia and, together with the Nagôs, was the prime mover in the early nineteenth-century Negro insurrections. The main cause of these insurrections, according to Ramos, was religious, having its foundations in the Islamic urge to *guerra santa* (holy war).[21] Moslem influence was present not only among the Hausa, but also in almost all the Sudanese Negroes, apart from those in the Guiné area.

Southey remarked that, in the seventeenth century, a traveller in Bahia 'might have supposed himself in Negroland',[22] so it is curious how the influence of Europe should have proved to be such a dominant one.

Large numbers of Portuguese immigrants belonged to the artisan class or came from small fishing communities, and Ott shows from researches in the public archives of Salvador[23] that the majority of these immigrants came originally from the northern province of Entre Douro e Minho, immigration from the south being much less considerable. The main attraction held by emigration was the hope of a better life and quickly accumulated wealth set against the over-exploited and fairly densely populated poor agricultural area in which they lived in Portugal. Emigration from this province became so great that, at one point in the eighteenth century, the Portuguese government issued orders to turn back ships of immigrants on arrival in Bahia. However, as Ott points out, the ships docked with only children and old people on board, the younger people, undoubtedly forewarned, having already disembarked on beaches above the entrance to the bay.[24]

Portuguese Catholicism was for centuries deeply imbued with countless pagan survivals which had become incorporated into the Christian year and practice. This trend was, and is still, particularly strong in the north of Portugal and in the bordering Spanish province of Galicia. Countless researchers have testified to the modern survival of semi-pagan practices in these areas.[25] The early Portuguese emigrants left a country in the grip of the Inquisition and a continent in the midst of widespread witch trials, with a general atmosphere of suspicion towards the superstition and superstitious practices which were so integral a part of the average peasant's life. These traditions were thus imported into Brazil along with the more orthodox forms of Catholicism, of which the Jesuit Order was the principal representative.

However, beliefs in certain semi-pagan practices and the propagation of rituals associated with these practices, if long since fused with Catholicism, were not solely restricted to the artisan classes, but also permeated the higher levels of society, so that the new aristocracy, the *senhores de engenho* (sugar-plantation owners), were also affected by them. It was inevitable that European folk practices should be adopted, especially in the field of medicine, in a society that was strictly divided between white masters and black slaves. The phenomenon of the power of 'white man's magic' is one that is very familiar and must have wielded great influence among the slaves of the colony.

Moreover, immigration from Portugal and from other European countries has been constant right up to the present day, and this has meant that European practices in Brazil have been undergoing a constant process of renewal. After 1930, restrictions were put on the naturalization of foreigners and a quota system introduced for all immigrants except the Portuguese:

In the 150 years up to 1969 Portugal contributed 1.8 million people to Brazil's population, against 1.6 million from Italy, 0.7 million from Spain, 0.3 million from Japan and 0.2 million from Germany.[26]

The 1974 figures on Portuguese immigration, however, show a drop in numbers, though this may change as Brazil's recent economic boom develops further:

In 1972, for the first time in over half a century, the Portuguese were not the largest immigrant group entering Brazil. The most numerous were the Koreans (1,895), followed by the Portuguese (807), with Americans third (675).[27]

Another element that has been introduced into the religious structure of Brazil comparatively recently is Spiritism.[28] The works of Léon Hippolyte Dénisart Rivail (1804–69), published under the pseudonym Allan Kardec, given to him by his spirit guide, rapidly gained popularity in Brazil.[29]

The long-established tradition in Brazil of Afro-European thaumaturgy was the principal factor in contributing towards the acceptance of Spiritism in the 1870s and in giving it the firm foothold which it enjoys today. It appeals to all social groups, but appears to tend towards merging most easily with African traditions among the lower social strata, while the higher echelons of society prefer to remain completely independent and practise the doctrines of Spiritism as laid down by Rivail and other writers without the presence of any outside influences.[30]

One of its principal doctrines is to practise charity and to cure illness which is believed to be caused by the actions of disembodied spirits. This is done through the assistance of *irmãos de luz* (spirits of light, i.e. those that are free from all evil) working through mediums who transmit beneficial *fluídos* (fluids) to the bodies of the faithful. Such *fluídos* are also known as *correntes* (currents), which flow, like an electric current, from one person to another.[31]

A federation of Spiritism was formed in 1884, since when it has ramified into many different associations which have established countless hospitals, clinics and assembly halls throughout the country, particularly in the south in São Paulo and Rio de Janeiro. According to Wilson:

. . . in the late 1950s there were some 7,000 spiritualist centres (of all kinds) in Rio de Janeiro alone, and one Catholic estimate for the archdiocese of Curitiba (capital of Paraná state) suggested that 40 per cent of the population was sympathetic to spiritualism.[32]

He goes on to quote Ferreria de Camargo:

They claimed to have provided hospital treatment for some 6,992 persons (compared with the Roman Catholic figure of 38,781, and the Protestant figure of 1,038), and they had provided assistance of some sort for 370,000 (compared to 503,000 persons assisted by the Catholics and 34,000 by the Protestants).

Such was the popularity of the Spiritism movement that in 1957 the Brazilian Post Office issued a postage stamp to mark the hundredth anniversary of Rivail's *Le Livre des esprits contenant les principes de la doctrine spirite.*[33]

The federation has continued to grow, and while no recent accurate figures are available, it is clear that it enjoys one of the largest followings of the major religious movements currently disseminated throughout Brazil.

CHAPTER III

THE PERSISTENCE AND DEVELOPMENT OF AFRICAN RELIGIONS

The colonists soon realized the importance to the African of his religion. Apart from providing a means of worship, it was looked upon by the Africans as a primary source of entertainment, and this quality it has retained in Brazil to this day. It was important, therefore, that the colonist should allow the practice of the cults to continue if he was to keep a high level of contentment among his work force. He managed to achieve this while keeping strictly to the requirements laid down by the Portuguese court and the Catholic Church, and merely insisted that the African should undergo baptism into the Catholic Church. Nothing more was required of him, apart from a short morning service on some plantations before the day's work began.[1] The Catholic Church's attitude was also one of mild tolerance. In fact, the development of African cults was openly encouraged, provided that the faithful switched allegiance from pagan deities to their Catholic counterparts.[2] All that this implied was a change of name, because the ceremonies themselves remained unchanged. More recently, however, this tolerance on the part of the authorities changed to open opposition. Various reports appeared in newspapers attacking African cults,[3] and the police made frequent raids when ceremonies were taking place and confiscated all objects sacred to the cult. It was confidently predicted that within a short while all the African religions in Brazil would disappear.[4] As the Brazilian economy expanded, however, especially during the decade following the revolution of 1964, it became clear to the authorities that such religions could be of tremendous use in the bid for development. First, they constituted an ideal tourist attraction (the main cult houses feature prominently on all the tourist propaganda issued by the state of Bahia, for example). But these religions could also be employed in the field of diplomacy, because they count Brazilians of African royal blood among their priestly hierarchies.[5] It is a fairly common occurrence now for a *mãe* or *pai de santo* to be sent by the Federal Government to Africa on what amounts to a royal visit. Such expeditions are given wide publicity in both continents and help to a very great extent to cement relations between the two.

The religion that the Africans brought with them is known in Bahia as

Candomblé,[6] in Recife as *Xangô*,[7] in Porto Alegre as *Pará*[8] and in Rio de Janeiro as *Macumba* and *Umbanda*.[9] The term *Macumba* is used to designate all the different African religions that came together in Rio de Janeiro, fused with all the other religious currents and took on an identity of their own in which characteristics borrowed from the Indian, the African and the European can be seen simultaneously. Outside Rio de Janeiro, the term *Macumba* is used in a slightly derogatory manner. Members of traditional cult houses in Bahia refer to members of fringe cult houses as people who *fazem Macumba* (literally 'do *Macumba*') (S.2), thereby implying not so much that the fringe cult houses are inferior as that they devote their attentions to evil ends. The term *macumbeiro* (one who practises *Macumba*) is extremely derogatory in Bahia and is used as a term of abuse.

The official religion of Brazil, Roman Catholicism, and *Candomblé* exist side by side in Bahia, and there is, on an official level at least, very little communication between the two.[10] *Candomblé* followers may be practising Catholics and may be seen at church on Sundays, but members of the priestly hierarchy confine their religious observances strictly within the walls of their cult house (I.2 and *passim*). Similarly, Catholic priests appear to have made few, if any, friends among the followers of *Candomblé*. The two religions rarely overlap on an official level, but on an unofficial level there have been marked movements towards syncretism, principally because on the surface there are striking similarities between the two. All the major Catholic saints find their counterparts in the Yoruba pantheon of deities (known as *orixás*), and so do God the Father and God the Son, though the third person of the Trinity is strangely lacking. Table 1 contains the names of the most common *orixás* with their Catholic counterparts.

Some of the connections between *orixás* and Catholic saints are obvious: Naná, the Old Matriarch, should clearly be linked with Saint Anne, the mother of the Blessed Virgin Mary; Omolú, the god of smallpox, is linked with Saints Lazarus and Roche; Oxossi, the god of the hunt, with Saint George, who killed a dragon, and so on. Others are less obvious, but there is always some overlap between the myth surrounding the African deity and the hagiographical background of the Catholic saint that justifies their being connected. Ogun, for example, is the god of war and he carries a sword with which he can *abrir caminhos*, literally 'open the ways', and, by extension, 'resolve difficulties', so he has become linked with Saint Anthony, patron of lost property. The African deity is

Table 1. The names of the most common *orixás* with their Catholic counterparts.

Orixá	*Domain*	*Catholic Equivalent*
Olorun	Father	God the Father
Oxalá	Son	Jesus Christ
Yemanjá	Salt water Fertility	Virgin Mary
Oxun	Fresh water Fertility	Virgin Mary
Naná	Old Matriarch	Saint Anne
Omolú (also known as Obaluayé, Abaluayé)	Disease, particularly smallpox	Saints Lazarus, Roche
Ogun	War	Saint Anthony
Oxossi	Hunt	Saint George
Yansan	Thunderbolt	Saint Barbara
Xangô	Thunder	Saint Jerome
Exú	Mischief	Devil

honoured on the feast day ascribed to his Catholic counterpart, and individual cult houses are dedicated to a particular deity in the same way as churches have their individual patrons. But here the syncretism ends. Ritual inside the traditional *Candomblé* cult houses contains no borrowings whatsoever from Catholic ritual and has remained purely African, the language of the ceremonies and incantations being the common language (Nagô) of the original Yoruba-speaking tribes in Africa;[11] and the ritual itself is identical to that currently practised in Africa.

The word *Candomblé* is Yoruba in origin and its true meaning is obscure.[12] *Candomblé* priests translate it into Portuguese as *brincadeira*, meaning literally a 'game', but this links it semantically with *brincar*, 'to jump'.[13] It refers particularly to the dancing that takes place on important feasts, during the course of which the *orixás* take possession of their followers, this occurrence being known as *montar a cavalo* ('riding a horse'). The word *orixá* has been loosely translated into Portuguese as *santo* (saint) and *guía* (guide). But it is also more commonly referred to as *dono da cabeça* ('owner of the head'), this being a direct translation of the Yoruba (*ori* = head, *xá* = owner). The *orixá*, therefore, actually owns the head of the person he chooses to follow him, according to Yoruba belief.

The conditions of choice are governed by a variety of factors: Omolú, the smallpox god, is automatically considered the owner of the head of one who has had that or any other skin disease. But usually a person's physical and psychological characteristics go towards determining which of the *orixás* he belongs to. A person with a look that reflects courage, stubbornness or determination will often belong to Ogun, god of war, or Yansan, goddess of the thunderbolt, who is also linked to war, and she carries a sword. She is the only *orixá* who, according to myth, is able to repel the spirits of the dead, known as *egun*.[14] Intelligence is associated with Oxossi, the hunter, always alert and lively; beauty, coupled with a gentle nature, links one to *as aguas* (the waters), i.e. the goddesses of water, Yemanjá and Oxun. It is not always the case that a man should belong automatically to a male *orixá* or vice versa, nor can it be proved that homosexuals show a tendency to belong to *orixás* of the opposite sex. The distinctions between characters go further than this, and it is usually the case that a person will reflect the characteristics of more than one *orixá*. Yemanjá and Oxun are linked since they both emanate from the waters and represent similar things, but a person who belongs primarily to Oxun will also show signs of being close to Oxossi, it being firmly established in the myths and legends that the two *orixás* were in love with each other.[15] In the same way, one who belongs to Oxun is not likely to be inclined at the same time towards Obá,[16] because they were both, in the myths, wives of Xangô, and the one was constantly fighting with the other.[17]

It used to be the practice (though this is now a fairly rare occurrence and would be restricted only to the traditional cult houses) for a man to consult the priest at the head of his *seita* (sect) as to the advisability or otherwise of his marrying a particular girl, it being very important, for reasons already given, that he should not marry one whose *orixá* would be incompatible with his own (S.4, C.1, C.5). It is clear that the determination of a person's *orixá* is very closely governed by his character and that the main qualification of a *mãe* or *pai de santo* should be good and accurate judgement of character. One *mãe de santo* (C.6) admitted that she was not normally over-fond of people who belong to Yansan, but was quick to add that this was based on her own assumption that people belonging to Yansan tend to have certain characteristics that she found particularly displeasing. It was not based on any lack of respect for the *orixá* concerned. Fundamental to *Candomblé*, therefore, is the notion that a person's *orixá* is determined by character—an *orixá* will only try to own the head of one who is compatible with himself or herself. It follows that, in the process of curing, the intercession of a particular *orixá* will be requested for assistance if the need arises. Yemanjá and Oxun will come to the aid of a man suffering from unrequited love, for example, while Yansan, once heard described as a *mulher macha* ('virile woman') (I.2) – the *orixá* who in the myths overcame the spirits of the dead – will succour those who are seriously ill.

In addition to this, each *orixá* has control over certain parts of the body, and an *orixá* may, by extension, be responsible for the malfunctioning of that part under his control, while remaining the chief means by which the cure may be effected.[18] The part of the body to which the *orixá* is linked is determined to a certain measure by myth, but particularly by logical association. Hence Exú, the mischief maker and guardian of all entrances and thoroughfares, looks after all the orifices of the body. Many *seitas* shun any association with him for the purpose of curing, though he is most important and powerful, and fundamental to the smooth running of every ceremony. This particular aspect can be seen most clearly by reference to Table 2. The colour associated with each of the main *orixás* is included.

Table 2. The areas of the human body controlled by *orixás*

Orixá	*Area of Control*	*Colour*
Oxalá	Head	White
Yemanjá	Childbirth Female sexual organs Stomach	Pink/white/light blue
Oxun	Childbirth Female sexual organs Stomach	Yellow
Xangô	Fever	Red and white
Naná	Rheumatic pains Skin diseases—linked with Omolú because of her great age	White/blue
Omolú	Skin diseases of all kinds, particularly smallpox, elephantiasis	Red and black
Ogun	Orifices of the body Procreation	Dark blue
Oxossi	Sterility Mental derangement	Green
Yansan	Fever	Red
Exú	Orifices of the body	Red and black

Periods of initiation into the religion vary considerably from one cult house to another. Traditionally, the candidate was expected to remain apart from other members of the cult house and from all family and friends for periods often exceeding one year. One of the *pais de santo* in Bahia recalled having spent fifteen months in isolation during his period of initiation, but nowadays three or four weeks is common (S.4). Traditional houses frown upon such short periods and declare that it is impossible to teach the initiate all that is necessary in that time. Indeed, this constitutes the main reason for the decline of the spoken African language in fringe cult houses, where it is considered sufficient to let the initiate proceed with just a smattering picked up by learning the incantations dedicated to the *orixá* in question. Traditional houses are particularly keen on the retention of the African language, and in one case in Cachoeira, the pertinent African language was spoken whenever children were present so as to give them as early a grounding in it as possible (C.1).

Initiation takes place particularly in the *ile orixá*, known in the vernacular as the *camarinha* (small room). The candidate will spend whatever period of time the high priest deems necessary in this room, in a state of semi-trance, known as *eré*.[19] *Eré* marks the intermediary stage between the normal and the ecstatic state, i.e. it is a stage somewhere between total possession by the *orixá* and a state of normality. Mediums in *eré* trances reveal a state of calm, childish ecstasy and act just like children. The twin *orixás*, known as Ibeji, particularly favour the *eré* trance state, and it is extremely common to see small altars erected in honour of the Ibeji in the bedrooms of children from all social strata.[20]

During the period of initiation, the candidate learns things of fundamental importance with regard to his future relationship with his *orixá*. Apart from the ritual language, he learns the incantations and drum rhythms associated with his *orixá* and a whole series of sung prayers known as *ingolosí* which are sung at specific times during the day or on specific ritual occasions by those who actually live in the cult house. The candidate also learns a certain amount about the ritual use of herbs. Herbs constitute a most important aspect of the *Candomblé* religion, and the candidate for initiation must learn which specific herbs belong to his *orixá* – but here his or her instruction may end because the secrets of the herbs are jealously guarded by the priestly hierarchy. The ultimate source of information is the *mãe* or *pai de santo*, who, ideally, pass down knowledge to their successors, a process, however, that can be interrupted by an untimely death, in which case the secret is lost for ever.

Herbs enter into all the main rituals. The candidate for initiation takes regular *banhos* (baths) called *abó* or *amasi*, and comes to relate the smell of these baths so automatically to the trance state that after initiation the smell of an *abó* or *amasi* mixture is sufficient to bring on a state of trance.[21] The candidate sleeps on a mat in the *ile orixá*, underneath which are specific combinations of certain herbs relevant to the *orixá* in question. After initiation, members are eligible to undergo other rituals, such as *obi* and *bori*,[22] in both of which herbs play an important part. Once a year the drums are 'fed' with herbs by having a herbal solution together with the blood of a sacrificial animal poured over them.

Due homage and respect are paid to dead members of Yoruba cult houses (known as the *egun*), and an exclusive cult of the dead is practised on the island of Itaparica, situated west of Salvador in the bay.[23]

Comments so far on *Candomblé* have in the main been restricted to the traditional cult houses in Bahia, of which there are very few left.[24] There is, on the other hand, a considerable number of houses in Bahia which have followed the example of the south of Brazil and accepted the influence of other religious movements. The African religions have been remodelled in such a way that they contain borrowings from Europe, to a lesser extent from the indigenous people of Brazil (Indians of Tupi stock), and from the relatively modern movement known as Spiritism.

The Brazilian Indian, although off the plantations, had left his mark firmly imprinted on Brazilian society, and the worship of Tupi spirits through a ritualistic framework based on *Candomblé* developed slowly at first, and then with great impetus in line with the nationalistic drives of the 1920s and 1930s when Brazil began to look in earnest to its indigenous heritage for most forms of artistic inspiration.[25] Spirits from the forest were seen more and more frequently in *Candomblé* cult houses, and now it is only the very few traditional houses that continue to ban the Indian spirits (known as *caboclos*) from mixing with their African counterparts. *Caboclo* spirits have been identified with various tribes of the Tupi stock,[26] and their names are always in either Tupi or Portuguese, e.g. Tupinambá, Maiongá, Jurema, Pedra Preta, Paraguaçú, Pedra Verde, Sete Flechas, Boiadeiro, Sultão das Matas, Janaina, Sete Estrelas, etc.

Candomblé de caboclo[27] enjoys its popularity for a number of reasons, the main one being that it is considerably easier for the faithful adequately to serve a *caboclo* spirit than an African *orixá*. The period of seclusion during initiation does not need to be nearly so long in that the *caboclo* incantations are almost always in Portuguese and *caboclo* cult houses use

Portuguese exclusively during rituals.[28] Some of the incantations, however, do contain some smatterings of African languages resulting in the curious occurrence of a Brazilian Indian spirit being praised in a mixture of an African language and Portuguese. Periodically there occurs in the incantations reference to a mysterious land called Aruanda which has become the lost paradise both for Africans and Indians.[29] Aruanda is, in fact, Luanda, the port on the coast of Angola, which passed into Afro-Brazilian folklore as a lost paradise in that it was the last place in Africa which many a slave had sight of as his ship started its journey across the Atlantic. It is typical of *Candomblé de caboclo* that *caboclo* spirits should also be assumed to have a connection with Luanda.

The *caboclo* spirits are also considerably less exigent than the African *orixás*, hence it is much easier for the faithful to fulfil their obligations.[30] The African *orixás*, for example, when they take possession of their followers, must be clothed in an elaborate costume which is provided by the *filhas de santo* at considerable expense, whereas the *caboclo* usually requires no more by way of a costume than a leather jacket and hat (Boiadeiro), or simply a feathered headdress and a lighted cigar.

It is curious how the *caboclos* have syncretized only with African deities and not with their Catholic counterparts.[31] Whereas it is common to hear Janaina referred to as *a mesma que Yemanjá* ('the same as Yemanjá'), it is extremely rare to hear Janaina related directly to the Catholic Virgin Mary. *Candomblé de caboclo* as an organized religion only emerged comparatively recently and has never been exposed to the Christianizing influence which predominated on the early sugar plantations, hence it has tended to emulate its African rather than Christian precursors. The influence of Spiritism (as opposed to Catholicism) has also been very marked, and much of *caboclo* terminology finds its origins in Spiritism.

All these elements, African *Candomblé*, the worship of Indian spirits, European popular beliefs and Spiritism, have come together under the generic title of *Candomblé de caboclo*, and it is certainly this type of *Candomblé* that predominates in Bahia today. *Candomblé de caboclo* is still mostly based on African and Tupi-inspired tradition although it is clear that Spiritism is gaining an ever-increasing hold. This may be due to the fact that Spiritism is a more intellectual movement that brings with it a prestige value and other refinements that the other religions are considered not to have. A number of informants mentioned that they felt considerably more at ease offering their services as mediums at a *sessão espírita* (spirit session, *séance*) than at a *Candomblé* ritual, in that the mediums at a *sessão* sit at a table and do not indulge in the sometimes frenzied and ungainly dancing in which they might otherwise participate. The traditional *seitas* fulfil a relatively minor role and cater for the needs of a very small number of people in comparison with the enormous following enjoyed by the *Candomblé de caboclo*.

Candomblé de caboclo as described above does not necessarily have to be a very organized affair, nor does it have to take place strictly within the walls of a consecrated cult house. People living in a normal dwelling house can set themselves up as *mães* or *pais de santo*, do secular work during the day and attend to the needs of the local community in their spare time. It is not at all important for them to have the trimmings usually associated with traditional houses. The reason for this is a purely financial one. People in poor suburbs of towns in remote areas do not have the wherewithal to establish themselves in houses which adequately fulfil all the conditions required by tradition. The result of this is that these fringe houses do not have to respect the ritual calendar. They can hold a *Candomblé* whenever they want to, and so it is fairly common, for example, for a *Candomblé* to be held to celebrate someone's birthday (I.3, I.6). In this way, the ritual fulfils its true function as a *brincadeira*, a game, played for the sake of enjoyment during leisure hours.

The main function of the *pai* or *mãe de santo*, other than that of administrative head of a cult house, is to advise and to cure, and all *pais* and *mães de santo* interviewed used the terms *curandeiro* and *curandeirismo* (folk doctor, folk medicine) when describing their functions. This is the case both in traditional and *caboclo* houses, and in the majority of instances the *pai* or *mãe* only deals personally with a member of the congregation when that member has a problem to solve.

The distinction between someone with a particular personal problem and someone who is ill and in need of a cure is a very fine one. A *pai* or *mãe de santo* may attribute a personal tragedy (such as the loss of a child) and a serious illness (such as elephantiasis) to the machinations of the same evil spirit. Everyday problems and specific illnesses tend to be placed under the one generic term 'indisposition', and invariably the same remedies are applied with more or less emphasis to indispositions at both ends of the spectrum. This does not mean to say that any isolated accident is automatically attributed to an evil force, though some cult members would readily say that this was the case (I.1, I.3, I.8, C.7, C.15, S.1).[32] However, an accident is always attributed to an evil force in the event of the victim's health deteriorating considerably subsequent to the accident.

All forms of indisposition, therefore, fall into two distinct categories in that they can be due to purely natural causes, or to a mysterious force known as *influência ruim* (bad influence). This *influência ruim* can either be deliberately inflicted by one individual on another, in which case it is called the evil eye (*mau de olho*), or it can arrive literally on the ill wind, in which case it is known as the *ar* or *moléstia do ar*. In this latter instance, no malice between individuals is involved in that the ill wind brings with it certain misfortunes and it is just the unhappy chance of the individual concerned to be contaminated.[33] In both instances, however, there is the notion that the indisposition concerned is caused by the undesirable presence inside the body of a force of evil, and it will be noticed that methods of curing such indispositions show a common tendency to expel the force of evil by physically driving it out of the body. Such a method of cure is common in folk medicine throughout the world,[34] and it is for this reason that the *curandeiro* has traditionally been concerned more with the spirit world than the material. If illness is considered not in terms of bacteria or germs that can be destroyed by means of a chemical process, but in terms of some form of evil force that is lurking inside the body and stopping it functioning in the normal way, then the cure will have to be undertaken on the same plane. Doctors of medicine in the past were not doctors at all in the modern sense of the word, but priests, since the expulsion of spirits was a function which only a priest was equipped to perform. The term 'witchdoctor' is used loosely nowadays, but it does convey the notion of the medicine man being linked to the world of the spirits in order to be able to carry out his functions successfully. The *curandeiro* in Brazil fulfils similar functions in that he is almost always a priest, often, but not necessarily, at the head of a cult house, and his followers will consult him when they are ill and the nature of the illness is seen to be beyond the limitations of popular remedies. It is the priest who has it in his power successfully to grapple with evil forces and therefore, ultimately, to bring about a cure.

CHAPTER IV

HERBS [1]

The importance of plant lore in the religions of the north-east of Brazil has been stressed elsewhere,[2] and informants constantly expressed the idea that herbs are important not only in the day-to-day relationship between man and the gods, but also in healing. Within the framework of *Candomblé*, all herbs, plants and trees belong to specific gods and come under their control, in the same way as parts of the body. These enter into the composition of dishes prepared as offerings to them, and are particularly important as part of curing rituals. Whatever the ritual, both in traditional and non-traditional cult houses, herbs play an extremely significant role. If a particular leaf is not available locally, the interested party may travel miles to find it. C.5 recalled having travelled to Feira de Santana, a distance of approximately eighty kilometres, to find a leaf he required for a specific purpose. People travelling into the interior, or to a neighbouring town, will invariably be asked by *curandeiros* to look out for some specific herbs and bring them back on their return.

Bastide suggests that the main reason why some *orixás* are now no longer worshipped in Brazil is that the herbs related to their cult cannot be found there,[3] and an informant in Cachoeira (C.5), while explaining the virtues of the *acoco* tree, had to admit that the secret as to which of the *orixás* it belonged to had died with a *mãe de santo* a few years previously. A result of this is that the *acoco* is now considered to belong to all the *orixás* together. He spoke of the tree in terms of great awe and respect, and said that of all herbs and plants that enter into ritual, this tree was one of the most significant and powerful, and yet this extremely important detail had been lost for ever.

One of the extraordinary aspects of plant lore is that all plants have, without exception, some power which, provided the right conditions are adhered to, will fulfil a definite purpose. A ritual requiring the use of a specific herb not readily available can still be performed in cases of urgency by using some other similar herb. Many informants agreed that, under these circumstances, *qualquer erva serve* ('any herb will do'),[4] but the one specified by tradition remains the most effective.[5]

On arrival in Brazil, the African recognized many plants that were identical to ones that grew in Africa, and those plants that were not indigenous to Brazil but of great importance in religious ceremonies were transplanted from Africa, the most important example being the *dendê* palm, now prolific in the north-east. Much information concerning plants indigenous to Brazil was acquired from the Tupi Indians, with whom the early African slaves worked for a while on the plantations. Many indigenous plants have since become incorporated in the *Candomblé de caboclo*, and they are often recognizable by their Tupi/Portuguese names, e.g. *nicurí de caboclo*,[6] *folha de urubú*, *imbé*, etc. Some plants indigenous both to Africa and north-east Brazil have lost their African name in favour of the Tupi, though this occurrence is restricted mainly to the interior and to areas further north of the state of Bahia, particularly Amazonas, where the Indian influence is more marked. An example of this is *Petiveria alliacea* L., known in Salvador and Itaparica as *guiné*, but in Cachoeira and further inland and northwards as *tipí*.[7]

The Portuguese and African drew on each others' knowledge of plants to a very great extent, mainly in the bid to use herbs to cure disease in remote areas of the interior around the capital where there were no doctors. As a result, the majority of herbs bear Portuguese names, the use of African names being restricted to the very traditional cult houses. Some of the plants indigenous to both the tropics and to Europe bear names that link them particularly to Europe, despite the fact that they appear to have no function in European folk medicine, their use being restricted to *Candomblé* ritual. An example of this is *Leonurus sibiricus* L., known in Brazil as *cordão de São Francisco* (Friar's cord). Catholic-sounding names, such as this one, may find their origin in the activities of the early Jesuit missionaries. Certainly, in the case of *Scoparia dulcis* L., the popular names in Brazil and Peru are virtually identical in meaning, the Brazilian version being *vassourinha* (small broom) and the Peruvian *escobilla del Peru* (small broom of Peru).[8]

Other herbs found in both Brazil and Europe have continued to be used according to past and present European tradition, while retaining their function in the context of African religious ritual. It is popularly believed in Brazil that anyone passing near a bush of *alecrim* (rosemary) should stop and savour its scent, and this custom is based on a considerably older Portuguese tradition, as shown in the following refrain from Vila Nova de Gaia:

> Whoever passed by the rosemary
> And did not smell it,

If he was ill
Became worse![9]

It is still used on haystacks and in grain barns in Galicia as a means of protection (G.2).

Arruda (rue), a most popular and important herb in Brazil, was used in ancient Greece and Rome as an amulet to protect against bad business and contagious illnesses, and is still highly esteemed by the Arabs for having been so favoured by Mohammed.[10] Rojas' great Spanish dialogue novel, *La Celestina*, which first appeared in 1499, bears witness to this herb's historical popularity in Europe: La Celestina herself is described as *mas conoscida (es esta vieja) que la ruda* (better known (is this old woman) than rue.) (Act IV). Its transition to the New World and subsequent popularity there is borne out by Debret's picture of *arruda* sellers drawn during his visit to Brazil in the early nineteenth century.[11] The following refrain from Barroso (Portugal) shows its importance as an amulet for protecting against evil:

Eighteen thousand sorcerers
I am not frightened of them.
I have a cross of rue,
On the crown of my head.[12]

The external appearance and physical composition of certain leaves correspond to a large extent with the personality of the *orixá* to whom they belong. Leaves fall into two main categories: *folhas bravas* (bold leaves) and *folhas finas* (delicate leaves), and as a broad rule *folhas bravas* tend to belong to masculine *orixás* who are stubborn, warlike or generally extrovert, while the *folhas finas* belong to *as águas* (the waters), i.e. Yemanjá, Oxun or Naná.[13] Yansan belongs to the former category in that she is the strong-minded, extrovert female *orixá* with many masculine characteristics.[14]

The principal leaves that belong to Ogun and Oxossi (gods of war and the hunt respectively) are *espada de Ogun* and *espada de Oxossi*. They are both very similar in shape and colour (green, and green and yellow respectively) and vaguely resemble drawn swords, hence are both very commonly seen standing in vases in people's houses or growing in pots at the entrance to protect the house from any evil that might try to enter it. An *espada de Ogun* was seen in a taxi in Salvador to protect the driver from assault. A brothel in Cachoeira had both plants growing at the entrance and a leaf from each pinned in the shape of a cross on the wall of the hall. Yansan's principal leaf is roughly the same shape, but smaller, and is reddish purple in colour.[15]

In contrast, however, certain delicate herbs (*folhas finas*) wilt in the presence of evil. *Vassourinha de Nossa Senhora*, when used to *rezar*[16] the evil eye, wilts completely during the ritual, which normally lasts only a few minutes, as the evil in the patient passes into it; and *avenca* and *macaça* bushes will wilt if a victim of the evil eye approaches them.[17] Another curious detail concerning *avenca and macaça* plants is that they must be looked after by only one person, otherwise they will die.

Opinions concerning the use of herbs vary radically from one *seita* to another, depending on the part of Africa from which they originated. Ultimately, the secret of the herbs in traditional *seitas* rests with the *pai* or *mãe de santo* concerned, and he or she will ensure that the laws governing their use are strictly adhered to. One of the features about *Candomblé de caboclo*, however, is that while herbs remain of the utmost importance in all rituals, the laws governing their use are extremely flexible. For example, a *Candomblé de caboclo* priest might cultivate some herbs in the land adjoining his house, though traditional houses abhor this practice and insist that if a herb is to be effective, it must be found growing wild in the jungle.[18] Often opinions concerning one particular herb or group of herbs vary so considerably that it is extremely difficult to come to any definite conclusion with regard to their use. One particularly salient example is the use of herbs belonging to Exú. Some *caboclo* priests use these herbs a lot since they feel that Exú has it in his power to deal with the most ferocious evil spirits. This is quite rare, however, and the majority of priests shun herbs that belong to Exú and take the view that, if the patient is possessed by Exú, herbs belonging to Exú should not be used in the cure. Such an attitude demonstrates how Exú's traditional link with the Catholic devil can be taken to extremes in certain circumstances. This does not imply, however, that these houses never resort to Exú for assistance. They do, but only in the context of specific rituals that take the form of returning evil forces to the person who originally sent them. If the doer of evil is known to the priest or the patient, then his evil force can be reversed and sent back to him. This would be done with materials that belong specifically to Exú, and such materials must be handled with extreme care and subjected to very special treatment.[19]

The picking of leaves and the gathering of seeds and nuts for curing is governed by a number of taboos, and these, with slight variations, appear to be standard to all *seitas*, both traditional and otherwise. The observance of taboos is of primary importance in that they serve to endow the herb with a special power, herbs that are picked without the observance of taboos being considered powerless.[20]

Usually, the person collecting the plant should be ritually pure, and this implies that he or she should have taken some form of bath, either herbal or otherwise, depending on the individual and the circumstances, after sexual relations, menstruation and so on. A herb that is picked when the body is ritually soiled (*corpo sujo*) is rendered worthless.[21]

It is considered imperative to ask permission (*pedir permissão*) from the relevant *orixá* before plucking any leaf growing wild in the jungle. In *caboclo* houses, this implies merely clapping the hands softly three times over the bush in question and saying three times *dá licença* ('please'), but in more traditional houses it is important to sing an incantation relevant to the *orixá* to whom the plant belongs.[22] Common to most *seitas* is the custom of leaving some small offering to the *caboclo* spirits of the jungle, or, in the case of traditional *seitas*, to Ossain, god of the forest. This offering usually takes the form of a small coin or a cigar.

In the case of particular herbs and seeds, great importance is placed on the direction in which they grow, on the sex of the person who may pick them, and whether or not they are picked with the left or right hand. *Cansanção*, for example, when picked with the left hand, can only be used for evil ends. The *fruta de São Cipriano* must be allowed to ripen and fall naturally from the tree. If it falls with the concave side facing upwards, it may be used as a powerful amulet to protect against the evil eye, but care should be taken to see that it is picked up by a man. If the convex side faces upwards, it may be used for evil, but only if picked up by a woman. Certain leaves that grow with the surface facing the sky must only be used for good purposes, while those that grow facing the ground must only be used for evil.

However, the purposes for which leaves or seeds may be used are not always governed by the direction in which they grow or the way they fall. It is of great importance that the picker of a leaf should have the intention of using it for good or evil firmly established in his mind before actually picking.[23] If by some chance a leaf picked for a specific evil purpose is not used, it may not under any circumstances be used for any other purpose. A leaf picked for an evil purpose remains powerful only in the context of evil and must not be used for good purposes. This notion of stating intention before undertaking such an act is fundamental to most ritual practices of this kind.

One of the principal rules governing the collection of herbs is the time of the day or night, or the date during the year on which they may be picked. Astrological factors such as the position of the sun, the phase of the moon and the season of the year govern the collection of certain herbs and seeds. A general rule is that herbs destined to be used for a good purpose should never be collected after sunset and before about 4 a.m., and if an urgent case arises whereby a ritual must be undertaken involving the use of herbs during the night, three pieces of charcoal must be used instead. It would appear that certain herbs retain their power only during the day, which implies that their power is linked in some way to the position of the sun. Certainly, when drying herbs for the purpose of making *pemba*,[24] it is advisable to dry them in the sun and not by artificial means (in the oven, for example) since it is believed that the sun imparts to them a special energy (I.2, C.5). One informant, C.10, stressed the importance of wearing light-coloured clothes when gathering herbs, and this in itself could be linked to associating the colour of the clothes of the picker with the light of the sun.

Traditionally, the rising sun and the waxing moon have been associated with the gathering of power and strength, while the setting sun and the waning moon imply the opposite. The full moon has a tremendous influence over the body, especially with regard to rheumatic pains, and bones that have once been broken are believed to give twinges of pain at the new moon and to stop hurting when the moon is on the wane (I.2, C.9).[25] Such a belief is reflected in the following ballad:

I buy snake's essence
And a measure of tobacco
To make an embrocation for my leg
Which hurts when the moon is full.[26]

It follows that the moon should be linked to man's vulnerability in catching diseases. Pliny tells of how '. . . the blood even of human beings increases and diminishes with its light', while other sources refer to how the moon can influence the increase or decrease of fever during the three days before and after the full moon, reaching the height of its powers at the equinox.[27]

It would appear that the virtue of a particular herb lies in direct relation both to seasonal variations and to specific astrological combinations. Hence, for example, the importance attached to collecting specific herbs on the eve of the feast of St John, a custom still followed not only in Brazil but in Spain and Portugal and in various other countries.[28] St John's feast day is significant in this context nowadays only in so far as it is on or around the ancient Midsummer Day,[29] which was the day when the season was considered to be at its most powerful.[30] Good Friday is another day which is considered most propitious for the collection of herbs, especially *dandá*, which takes on a special power to protect against the evil eye if picked on that day.

It follows that the time at which the seed of a plant is sown can be of equal significance, and for this reason the sowing of some plants is accompanied by a peculiar ritual. The *lança de Oxalá* should be sown on a Friday in the middle of a pentangle scratched on the ground.[31] Considerably more complex rituals are necessary in the case of the *acoco* seedling which should be covered every day at 6 p.m. with four brand-new high-quality sheets. C.5 actually went so far as to mention the brand name of the sheets which would be ideal for the purpose. The following morning at sunrise the sheets are lifted by four virgin girls. This day-to-day ritual continues until the seedling is about a foot high.[32]

The vast majority of herbs, however, are in constant use, and because they are considered to be more efficacious when employed freshly picked, are collected throughout the year. Such herbs only come under the influence of the sun and/or moon, and this accounts for the detailed instructions that must be adhered to when picking them. The moon must be in a specific phase, or the sun at a particular angle in the sky. Observation of the position of the sun has now been superseded to a great extent by the hours of the day, and hence, instead of it being specified that a herb be picked before sunrise, it is specified that it should be picked at around 4.30 a.m. The actual time when it may be picked is reduced to fairly narrow margins, as in the case of *betis cheiroso*, which may be picked only between 3 and 4 a.m. Further complications arise when a herb may only be picked when both the sun and the moon are in juxtaposition to each other, the position of the moon usually being judged by the state of the tides. Hence *salsa da praia* can only be picked between 4 and 5 a.m., and then only when the tide is coming in—a situation that occurs only rarely during the month. This practice is not restricted to African ritual and was common throughout medieval Europe.

Other herbs may only be picked on specific days of the week when the sun is in a specific position. This day is usually the one dedicated to the worship of the *orixá* to whom the herb happens to belong—hence *canela de velho* can only be picked on a Monday because that is the day dedicated to Omolú, who controls the plant.

Sometimes, though, the situation is complicated by the herb in question being ascribed divergent qualities at different times of the day so that it can belong to more than one *orixá* depending on the time of day it happens to be. This metamorphosis in character sometimes takes place during remarkably short periods of time, as, for example, in the case of *coerana*, which belongs either to Ogun, Yansan or Omolú between 4 and 9 a.m., and to Exú between 9 a.m. and midnight. Six o'clock in the morning and evening, and midday and midnight are times when no herb or leaf may be picked for good purposes (with the exception of *gameleira*), since these are the times when it is considered that evil forces are at their most powerful and herbs lose all their beneficial virtues.[33] The allegiance of some plants is momentarily changed at these times, as in the case of the *gameleira*, which normally belongs to Exú but every six hours comes under the control particularly of Omolú because those are the times when, according to one informant (C.2), *os espíritos maus descansam no pé da gameleira* ('the evil spirits rest in the *gameleira*'). Trees such as this are greatly feared mainly because of the link with Exú (*não gosto de trabalhar com ela*—'I don't like working with it' (I.2)), but if the leaves are picked at times when they belong to Omolú, they are considered an extremely powerful means of curing and are mixed with other herbs for fumigation and ritual baths.

It is clear, then, that, as the positions of the sun or moon change, so does the *orixá* to whom the herb belongs at different times of the day, and consequently the herb's sphere of influence is altered. Mention has already been made of how each *orixá* controls certain parts of the body so that the change in virtue of the herb corresponds to the different areas of control of each *orixá*. This is very much akin to the European idea of linking each herb to a planet and ascribing to it different virtues in accordance with the planet's position in relation to other planets in the universe.[34]

Similarly, in Brazil, it is believed that the position of the moon and the sun can have a marked effect on the sap of growing plants and that specific conjunctions of heavenly bodies produce situations whereby man becomes especially prone to specific diseases.[35] It would appear therefore that, as resistance to a disease diminishes, so certain herbs used to cure that disease are believed to increase in power. They are believed to become weaker in respect of one *orixá* and more powerful in respect of another as the day progresses (C.5, C.10, C.12).

It is a fact that in certain cases herbs belonging to one *orixá* are used to cure disorders in that part of the body over which the *orixá* has control. This is particularly the case concerning skin disorders and diseases that cause scabs to appear on the skin (smallpox, leprosy, etc.) and which come under the dominion of Omolú. Matters become more complex, however, when the cure for a particular disease requires the application of two or more herbs, but this must be based on empirical experience when it has been observed that symptoms of a specific nature coupled with other symptoms imply that the indisposition concerned comes within the area of control of two or more *orixás*, hence the application of further herbs. In the majority of cases, the *orixá* of the patient concerned will require that a sufficient quantity of the herbs under his control be included in any group because otherwise he will become displeased and hinder the process of the cure.

A man with a disorder that comes under the dominion of an *orixá* totally alien to his personality should be treated for that disorder with a preponderance of herbs belonging to his own *orixá* and with a certain number devoted to the *orixá* who has control over the disorder in question. Hence, in one case of leprosy encountered, the patient, who belonged to Yemanjá, had seven consecutive baths on seven consecutive days, each bath consisting of three herbs belonging to Omolú (god of skin diseases) and four or six belonging to Yemanjá and others (C.2).

The use of herbs in specific rituals, namely ritual baths (*banhos*), fumigation, the preparation of amulets and so forth, will be discussed in detail in subsequent chapters.

CHAPTER V

THE SACUDIDA (RITUAL BEATING)

As we have already seen (page 21), there is a common tendency in folk medicine to deal with forces of evil by physical means, and so, in the case of illness or mental disturbance, it is believed that the evil spirit must either be frightened away by a sound beating, as if it were a tangible entity, or else attracted into the instrument used in beating, which can then be broken and disposed of, carrying the evil with it. McKenzie (1927:84) testifies to this practice among the Yuruna Indians of Brazil:

Among the Yuruna Indians of Brazil the doctor violently rubs his sick people with a green twig all over the body. Having in this way caught the disease in the twig, he then carries it carefully outside, groaning heavily all the time and throws it away.

Akin to this practice, but more closely related to the idea of frightening away the spirit than that of attracting it and then destroying it, is that alluded to by Freyre among other tribes, of individuals flogging one another when sick.[1]

The African religions in Brazil contain a number of rituals that include flogging, and this is particularly apparent in the Yoruba *egun* cult festivals on the island of Itaparica where the *egun* (spirit of the dead) is kept away from onlookers by a priest who beats the ground in front of the spirit with a cane. The spirits are not evil as such, but they are greatly feared because they are believed to bring instant death to any living person they come in contact with through a desire to reincarnate themselves in a living body. Yoruba peoples in Africa today attribute many misfortunes and illnesses to the anger of the spirits of the dead.[2]

Beating with a stick is also an important aspect of the *quitanda* (market stall) ritual, another Yoruba legacy, in which the initiate enters the cult house bearing on her head a tray of fruit and clothes made during her seclusion, and beats with a stick those who try to steal anything off the tray. Here the initiate is emerging from a period of seclusion and is in an extremely vulnerable state, hence the importance attached to her beating off those who may look with envy upon the goods on display, thereby exposing her to the dangers of the evil eye.[3] In this case, however, it may be regarded as a preventive measure rather than the actual expulsion of recognized evil spirits.

The Europeans had a ritual similar to the indigenous and African ones just described in which forces of evil were frightened away, albeit in a much less strenuous fashion. Instead of sticks or twigs, they lightly brushed sprigs of specific leaves over the patient's body while reciting a prayer or charm, but more attention will be given to this in a subsequent chapter.[4] It is mentioned here just to demonstrate how members of all three cultures that came together in Brazil practised the custom of brushing or violently beating leaves or twigs against or near the body in order to drive away forces of evil. The term *sacudida* (a shaking) implies that a similar process is being enacted, for during a *sacudida*, certain leaves from certain plants are beaten violently against the patient to the accompaniment of certain prayers. As a result, all the evil forces are driven away.

There are around thirty leaves that may be employed for purposes of a *sacudida* (see Appendix One), and of these approximately seven are the ones most commonly employed. They are given in Table 3, together with the *orixá* or *orixás* who control them. It will be observed that they all come under the control of one or more of a group of five *orixás*, and it is significant that they should do so, because each of these *orixás* is particularly suited in his or her own way to overcome forces of evil of all kinds. Exú, the trickster god, syncretized in *Candomblé de caboclo* with the Catholic devil, guards all entrances, therefore all orifices in the human body that may have been penetrated by the force currently making the patient ill. He is also the *orixá* that must be satisfied by means of the sacrifice of an animal, or, more commonly, a small offering of food or a candle, before any ritual takes place, otherwise he will become angry and threaten to jeopardize the whole proceedings.[5]

Table 3. The most commonly used herbs in the *sacudida* with their *orixás*

Leaf	*Orixá*
aroeira	Exú, Omolú, Yansan, Oxossi
coerana	Omolú, Exú, Ogun, Yansan
espada de Ogun	Ogun
espada de Oxossi	Oxossi
espada de Yansan	Yansan
guiné	Omolú
Sao Gonçalinho	Oxossi, Omolú

An evil spirit that enters a person's body and makes him ill is often referred to as an *exú*. This evil spirit is considered to have been sent by an enemy through a ritual sacrifice or offering made by that enemy, and the cure often consists of making even larger gifts to Exú the *orixá* and requesting him to drive the evil away from the patient's body (C.1). In *caboclo* terms, he is looked upon as being a potential evil force that can be wooed to either side, hence he shares control of two of the most powerful and popular leaves used for *sacudidas*.

The other four *orixás* all have strong links through myths with death, and it is for this reason that evil spirits are frightened away by them. Oxossi, the hunter, and Ogun, the warrior, inflict death in the normal course of their duties, while Omolú, the god who brings smallpox, also has the power to kill. His drum rhythm is called in Yoruba *opanijẹ*, which means 'He kills someone and eats him', and similar themes relating to his power to kill emerge in the incantations dedicated to him.[6]

Yansan's assistance is requested especially in that she is the only *orixá* who can overcome death and who is capable of standing up to the *egun*. This ability to overcome death is alluded to in incantations dedicated to her, as in the following example collected in Cachoeira (C.7):

Oya Oya,[7] she is the mistress of the world. *Oya Oya*, Yansan overcame everything. *Oya Oya*, she is the mistress of the world. *Oya Oya*, Yansan overcame death.

Her fearlessness in the face of death is such that a certain amount of tact must be employed by the *curandeiro* when treating a patient who belongs to Yansan in that he should under no circumstances employ *coerana* in the *sacudida*. *Coerana* is believed to have power to frighten away the *egun*, and also spirits of the dead who like to linger near their relatives on earth and pester them in such a way as to make them become ill.[8] The leaf, which belongs in part to Yansan, may be used on anyone provided that Yansan is not his or her *orixá*, because she may become jealous and try to assert her superiority over the leaf at the expense of the patient's well-being (C.5).[9] I.2 and C.2, however, did not make this distinction.

The best times for a *sacudida* to take place are early in the morning, when the sun is gathering strength (I.2), or at sunset, *para que o sol leve tudo* ('so that the sun can take everything away') (C.2). The leaves must be freshly picked while observing all the taboos peculiar to each. Sometimes the herbs are dipped first into a bowl of salt water, but this is rare nowadays (C.1, C.5). Four small heaps of gunpowder are placed on pieces of paper around the patient, who must stand facing the open door so that the evil may leave the room easily (I.2, C.2). A candle is lit outside in the yard for Exú (I.2 and *passim*). The *curandeiro* takes a combination of three different plants and uses three sprigs of each, totalling nine sprigs. Sometimes, in very serious cases, the number of sprigs goes up to fourteen and twenty-one in total (I.2, C.1, C.2). The *curandeiro* starts hitting the patient about the neck with the leaves, and slowly works his way down to the feet. Every now and then he shakes the leaves in the direction of the open door as if shaking off any evil that may have passed on to them. Throughout the ritual the following prayers (usually in improvised forms) are said:

1 Senhor Ogun, with the powers that God gave you, with the sword that you carry, I ask you that you with these forces break the evil, the bad influences which may be in this person, and also the disturbances and malignant forces. I ask you to give strength to this person, break the force of the evil eye, in the name of our heavenly Father. In the name of Jesus. Ave Maria. Ogun *ye*, Ogun *ye*, Ogun *ye*.[10] [I.2]

2 O twenty-one Oguns, with your swords cut away all the evil that might be within this person. I implore all the *orixás* to help in this task. All are brothers. Help to break the forces, to cast out these radiations which are here. All the *orixás*, all the Oguns, the twenty-one Oguns, old Omolú, by the day that is today, my father Oxossi, I beg you to break the forces of these evil eyes, these bad influences, these false friends, in the name of our heavenly Father. Ogun *ye*, Ogun *ye*, Ogun *ye*.

3 I implore you, Senhor Ogun, that you cut away all the evil that is here, any person who might have an evil heart, any evil thought. Look after them. Break all these evil eyes.

In the case here cited, the leaves employed were *espada de Ogun*, *espada de Oxossi* and *São Gonçalinho*, and it is clear from the prayers that the *espadas* are believed actually to have the power of real swords, to cut the evil in half and break it, e.g. '*cut away* all the evil'. Qualities such as these are ascribed to a large number of leaves whose appearance is suggestive of implements associated with driving away evil by physical means and whose names imply that this is the most effective use to which they may be put.

When the leaves have been beaten all over the body, they are broken and thrown outside the door into the street. The *curandeiro* now lights each of the small heaps of gunpowder in turn, and as each heap explodes he stamps once with his left foot and pours water on the ashes saying, *O que apaga o fogo é agua* ('What extinguishes fire is water'). This is done in order to establish the *curandeiro*'s superiority over the spirit in question, for if he has the power to frighten away the spirit with fire, he shows himself to be doubly powerful if he can wield power over fire with water (I.2). The use of gunpowder in this way to frighten away forces of evil is extremely common in Brazil, and it can be readily purchased in markets and in chemist shops in the interior.

The final stage of the ritual is fumigation, which will be dealt with at length in the next chapter.

CHAPTER VI

FUMIGATION

Fumigation has played an important part in ritual throughout the world, its primary function in most cultures being to purify. Fumigation, conducted under the right conditions, will cleanse the air and the body of all evil forces that may affect health or general well-being, but it is also employed as an important constituent in most healing rituals.

The reason why it is used as a purifying agent is based on the notion that fire, the ultimate purifier, will, when in contact with specific ingredients, produce smoke that serves either to repel forces of evil or to attract forces of good. Smoke, together with the perfume that is part of it, is looked upon as being something which is esoteric, that cannot be grasped with the human hand and that establishes a link between the world of men and the world of the gods. The continued use of incense in fumigatory ritual in Europe most probably finds its origins in ancient Egyptian practice. Wallis Budge (1928:24) points out how incense, along with a number of other substances, was believed to be of divine origin, hence its use in ritual:

> On certain occasions SHU and TEFNUT weep, and when their tears reach the ground they sink into the earth and transform themselves into the plants from which incense is made.

Fire itself has a long history in folklore in that it serves to destroy all useless or evil things while opening the way for the beginning of a new and purer existence. Judas burning, which is closely linked to the fertility of crops,[1] or the burning of *fallas* (wax statues) in Valencia (Spain) and similar practices that take place about the time of the equinox, reflect this notion that fire destroys in order that something new may be created.[2] It is, then, associated with fertility and the notion of mystical rebirth in that it is always followed by the birth of a new season, a new state of affairs emerging out of the old. In Europe, particularly in Spain and Portugal, bonfires were lit close to the solstice[3] for specific purposes. Jumping over the fire was considered to remedy various conditions. Childless couples would jump over the fire so that it would frighten away the evil spirits that were preventing them from having children, and marriageable youths would do likewise to ensure gaining a partner in marriage. Proximity to fire also extended into the area of curing and preventing disease in that jumping over a bonfire was considered adequate protection against catching the plague, and the ashes of herbs both collected and burned on the night of the feast of St John could be used throughout the year for purposes of curing.[4]

Such practices are now only re-enacted in the Peninsula for amusement and for the sake of keeping up ancient traditions, but much of the solstice bonfire tradition has survived in Bahia, where it is faithfully re-enacted each year since a large proportion of the population continues to take such things seriously. Fire continues to play a particularly important part in Brazil in the field of curing. Maynard Araújo makes mention of a cure for impotence in men which consists of the patient making as if to sit on hot coals.[5] Sometimes the fire is expected sympathetically to take away the last vestiges of disease, as, for example, in the case of a cure for warts in which pieces of rock salt that have been rubbed over the wart are then thrown into the fire (I.1, I.7, C.7, C.13, C.15, S.5). In a cure for erysipelas, the mixture of water and oil in which herbs are steeped before being used to bless the patient is left in the hearth and allowed to dry out. It is believed that the illness will leave the patient's body at the same time (C.14). If it is essential to conduct a *reza*[6] at night, then it should be done near the fire or stove, or at least with a few hot coals in an empty censer placed near the patient (I.2, C.5). The cotton reel used to *rezar* a twisted ankle or pulled muscle is hung up over the fire or stove, presumably either to dry up the pain that has passed into it or to recharge it with new energy (I.2).

Traditional European solstice and equinox practices merged very smoothly with African and indigenous rituals that involved the use of fire. Fire plays an important role in Brazilian *Candomblé*, which has retained the traditional African method of testing whether or not a particular *orixá* is the correct one for an initiate by subjecting the initiate when possessed to the test of fire. If the initiate can swallow a live coal or expose his or her hands to flames without making any adverse reaction, this is taken as proof that the *orixá* in question is the correct one and that the trance is not being simulated.[7] João do Rio describes a fire test consisting of the initiate in question having hot oil poured over her head,[8] while in *Candomblé de caboclo* it is very common for the medium, once possessed, to place the lighted end of a cigar between his lips, or to set light to a heap of gunpowder in his outstretched palm to prove his power to the onlookers (I.2, I.3).

The idea that a good spirit in possession of or protecting a human being will not in any way be affected by contact with fire is countered by the notion that evil spirits are not only incapable of withstanding fire but may even be destroyed by it. This belief is very ancient and is still testified to in some countries during rituals involving people walking barefoot over hot coals or undergoing similar ordeals which appear to leave them unharmed. It is very strong in the Christian tradition, and it accounts for the custom that was prevalent in the past of subjecting condemned witches to burning at the stake so that the death of the body would be accompanied by the complete destruction of its evil soul.[9]

A number of *orixás* are linked through the myths to fire, hence a Xangô initiate must carry a live brazier on her head and undergo other fire tests because Xangô is the god of thunder and lightning and himself closely connected with fire.[10] Yansan, the goddess of the thunderbolt, is one of the wives of Xangô, and therefore also connected with fire. She has been adopted as patroness of Brazilian firemen, who carry her picture (usually that of her Catholic counterpart, Saint Barbara) in their fire engines. Ogun, the god of war and metal, is also very closely linked to fire because he presides over the smithy, where metal tools of all types are manufactured.[11] Exú, the trickster god, is the nearest in Africa to a fire god in that it was he who, at the beginning of time, brought the sun for the benefit of mankind, and hence is worshipped around the time of the solstice.[12] It is this link with fire that rendered his syncretism with the Catholic devil—always depicted against a background of hell-fire—the more acceptable to the early African slaves. Many of the herbs associated with Exú sting when touched and leave a burning sensation on the skin (the Portuguese *queimar*—to burn—being used to describe this).

The Brazilian Indian, too, ascribed miraculous powers to fire, seeing it as an agent that could be linked to fecundity and hence able to inflict a fundamental change on the objects with which it came into contact. Making fire by rubbing sticks together was looked on as being a representation of the sexual act,[13] while the process of cooking implied that a fundamental change of state was taking place. The food could be said to be leaving a profane state and becoming sacred.[14]

It is clear that the process of fumigation depends to a large extent on the combination of the powers of fire with the powers inherent in the substance being used to fumigate. Karsten mentions the importance of fumigation with tobacco and other herbs as a means of purification,[15] and Stade refers to the Tupinambá practice of fumigating the sacred *maracá* gourd rattles with tobacco before use.[16] Its main function, however, is that of repelling evil forces and leaving the object fumigated ritually clean and able to be used in dealings with the gods. Similarly, fumigation of this nature is used in curing rituals to drive away the forces of evil producing the disease. Purí-Coroado Indians who were ill were fumigated by their shamans with tobacco smoke as part of the process of curing,[17] and similar methods were used by the Tupinambá,[18] and still are used today by many Indians in the Amazon Basin.[19] Tobacco smoke is looked upon by them as being sacred, since it is a means of inducing in the smoker a state of ecstasy whereby he can be in direct communication with the gods and achieve a spiritual state superior to the normal physical state; hence, when it is blown over the patient, it will have added power. Tobacco is currently used in this way in *Candomblé de caboclo*, where it is common for the *orixá*, once manifested, to request a cigar and then puff smoke over anyone who approaches and consults him for a remedy for a specific complaint (I.2 and *passim*).

The smell of the substance used to fumigate is also of great importance because, clearly, if a substance has an attractive smell when burned, it will have a different function in fumigating ritual than a substance which has an unattractive smell. Substances employed for fumigation tend to fall quite easily into these two distinct categories, and it follows that malodorous substances are burned in order to repel undesirable forces which may be causing the indisposition in question, while sweet-smelling substances are burned in order to attract beneficent influences.[20] Thus garlic straw and dust picked up from a crossroads, powdered horn or hoof, manioc flour and similar materials are burned to repel forces of evil (*afastar*), while substances like incense, storax and sugar are employed to attract beneficent forces (*atrair*).

Animal excrement is an important agent in Brazil for repelling forces of evil, and its inherent power is to be found not so much in the unpleasant smell that it produces on burning as in the sacred quality attributed to dung in this and other cultures as a cleansing agent. Brazil has shown itself in recent years to be a watershed for different religious practices and rituals from all over the world, and has always been quick to assimilate new ideas coming in from outside. The sanctity of the cow is well known in Asia, and cow dung is commonly used as a means of purification:

Cows are sometimes said to be gods . . . Cow-dung, like the dung of any other animal, is intrinsically impure and can cause defilement—in fact it will defile a god; but it is pure relative to a mortal . . . the cow's most impure part is sufficiently pure relative even to a Brahmin priest to remove the latter's impurities.[21]

It is typical that, in Brazil, such a practice should be extended to include the excrement of other animals as well. If Spiritism can readily be incorporated under the cloak of *Candomblé*, it is only a short step to include the dog and other animals in the same category as the Asian sacred cow. Dog excrement is used extremely frequently in fumigation,[22] and it is also taken internally, infused with water, though *curandeiros* are careful to point out that under no circumstances should the patient learn precisely what the ingredients of the medicine are (I.2 and *passim*).[23] Elephant excrement appears to be considered powerful mainly because elephants are not indigenous to Brazil and hence the excrement acquires rarity value. Substances which are rare in Brazil, or which can only be found outside, are much sought after by *curandeiros* because they are attributed considerable power on account of their rarity. *Curandeiros* rely for their supplies of elephant excrement on the infrequent visits of travelling circuses, and it is significant that the use of elephant excrement is not known at all on the island of Itaparica, which was until fairly recently accessible only by canoe and small fishing boat.[24]

Other substances are used to repel forces of evil because they come from places associated with death (e.g. cemetery dirt), or because they are closely linked to a repulsive or dangerous animal. Hence the mud wall of an ants' nest or the wings of a cockroach may be included as ingredients.

Substances such as incense and storax have been used in fumigation to attract good in many different cultures for a very long time, and they feature prominently in medieval texts on occult practices.[25] More recent publications that rely heavily for their information on earlier texts also suggest the use of these ingredients. Reference is made particularly to the *Livro Antigo e Verdadeiro de São Cipriano* and the *Cruz de Caravaca*, both of which enjoy enormous sales in Brazil and have run to many impressions.[26]

Incense in particular is employed to attract good, but it is rarely used by itself and is more often employed in conjunction with other substances, particularly herbs.

Curandeiros prefer to make up their own mixtures for purposes of fumigation, but there is a wide selection of marketed varieties of herbs readily available in street markets for use in the house. These appear to be extremely popular and sell very well,[27] but they all come without exception from suppliers in the south of Brazil, particularly São Paulo and Rio de Janeiro.[28] Most stalls bought in bulk and packeted locally so as to include their own names on the packet, but all stall-owners admitted they would never impart such information to their customers (S.6, S.7, S.8, S.9, S.10). Stall-owners are regarded by the public as cheap *curandeiros* who fulfil rather the same function in *curandeirismo* as the chemist in modern medical practice.

Approximately 50 per cent of the marketed varieties have woodcuts on the packets showing a link between all the substances enclosed and an *orixá* who is either African or *caboclo*, but *curandeiros* who make up their own varieties emphasize that specific combinations of herbs need betray no affinity to any one *orixá*, apart from the ones who control each individual herb. It is impossible to analyse the precise herb content of marketed varieties because the different leaves have been crushed into such small pieces that they are quite unrecognizable, but most of the packets betray the same characteristic smell when burned. It would appear that the affinity to an *orixá* bears little or no relationship to the herbs employed in the vast majority of marketed varieties of fumigators, but that the name of the *orixá* is included on the packet to cater for the needs of those who only like to work with substances that belong exclusively to or are associated with their individual *orixá*. Such feelings of loyalty to one's personal *orixá* are very typical.

Sometimes, however, the name of the variety will not include the name of an *orixá*, but will state the definite purpose for which the fumigator should be used, i.e. *Desmancha Tudo* ('destroy everything'); *Quebra Feitiço* ('spell breaker'); *Tira Mofina* ('get rid of misery'); *Vence Tudo* ('overcome everything'); *Tira Teima* ('get rid of obstinacy'); and it will be observed that all these names betray a preoccupation with the same thing—namely, overcoming the force of evil causing the indisposition in question.

A large number of the packets contain many allusions to countries outside the Iberian peninsula and the West Coast of Africa, mainly in order to mention the exotic for the sake of making the substance in question appear the more powerful. Hence a packet with a woodcut of Saint Roche calls him *São Roque de Ceilão* (of Ceylon), while other packets describe their contents as being

prepared with all requisites from Indo-African science; Made with material and plants imported directly from the African and Indian coasts;

to achieve everything desired by the occult persons of Indian science; the product of Egypt which symbolizes the gods of ancient Egypt, and the protector of the dead, Osiris. Oriental product . . .

Such mention of India and the Egyptian god Osiris is more characteristic of southern Brazilian *Macumba*, which has more readily accepted influence from religions other than the traditional European, African and indigenous ones. Binon Cossard suggests that this movement in Rio de Janeiro away from a preoccupation with things that are legitimately African reflects an unconscious desire on the part of the Brazilian lower classes, who are usually dark-skinned, to go up the social ladder towards the position of the middle- or upper-class white.[29] I feel that this is not necessarily the case, however, in Bahia, where the mention of India or Egypt on a packet contributes more to the product's likely efficacy.

At times, a packet manufactured in the south of Brazil and bearing the local Bahia distributor's stamp will contain information on the label which should be totally unacceptable in Bahia, even in the more flexible *Candomblé de caboclo* cult houses. Fumigators bearing the name of St George are often allied as well to Ogun, a characteristic of *Macumba*, whereas in Bahia Saint George is nowadays only related to Oxossi.[30] Such obvious dichotomies do not appear to matter, and informants all agreed that the 'mistake' was just a characteristic of *Macumba*, the fumigator itself being considered as worth while as any other.

There is much more demand for fumigators that are home made than for the marketed varieties, and this is based not so much on an essential conservatism as on what people regard as the dubious efficacity of the contents of the packet. The herbs and other ingredients are so unrecognizable that there is a genuine fear of there being something in the mixture which may ultimately do more harm than good. At least with the home-made varieties of fumigator people know precisely what the ingredients are, and the main ingredient is usually one or more herbs.

The number of herbs that may be used for fumigation is quite large (approximately 40 per cent of those quoted in Appendix One), but only a very few of these are, in fact, used all the time. These are shown in Table 4, together with the *orixás* to whom each belongs. It will be noted that those herbs used to repel forces of evil belong to Ogun, Yansan or Omolú, the first two of whom are *orixás* associated with physical power. They both carry a sword with which they are able to overcome most

Table 4. Attributes of the most common herbs used in fumigation, with their *orixás*.

Attract		*Repel*	
Herb	*Orixá*	*Herb*	*Orixá*
alfazema (leaf) picked before midday	Oxun Yemanjá	*alfazema* (leaf and seed) picked after sunset	Yansan
arruda	Yansan	*arruda*	Yansan/Omolú
capim de caboclo	Yansan	*abre caminhos*	Ogun
manjericão	Oxun Yemanjá/Naná/ Oxalá	*tira teima*	Ogun
		vencetudo	Ogun

difficulties with ease. Those herbs associated with Ogun reveal this quality in their names, which contain references to physical intervention on the part of the *orixá*: *abre caminhos* ('open the ways'); *tira teima* ('get rid of obstinacy'); *vencetudo* ('overcome everything'). Omolú's ability to repel and the reasons for it have already been discussed.[31]

Those herbs used to attract good belong to Oxun, Yemanjá, Naná, Oxalá and Yansan, and all these *orixás*, with the exception of Yansan, are at first sight associated with gentleness, calm and other similar characteristics which are more suitable for attracting good forces than expelling evil ones. Yansan, however, may enter into this category in that she has a double-sided character. Usually she is the archetype of impetuous, domineering women, but she does have a side to her character which is more feminine and more gentle. Her *filhas de santo* quite readily put themselves into these two different categories, the more extrovert ones saying that they belong to *Yansan pé de abano* (Yansan of the fan-shaped foot) and the less extrovert ones claiming allegiance to *Yansan do pé lavado* (Yansan of the washed foot). Yansan is not alone among the *orixás* in having these two sides to her character, Yemanjá and Oxun particularly standing out as the *orixás* usually associated with beauty and equilibrium, but also with the primeval forces associated with the sea and with rivers. Yemanjá, goddess of salt water, is related in myths to the life-giving principle behind all living things in that it was she who gave birth to all the other *orixás*.[32] Oxun, goddess of fresh water, is very close to her, and they are often depicted in statues or pictures as erotic mermaids or finely clad goddesses emerging from the sea with accentuated breasts and hips to underline their importance as fertility figures. Stories about the faithful to their cult are riddled with instances of self-sacrifice, or of the goddess herself claiming her son or daughter.[33] There is, therefore, an extremely forceful side to their characters, and for this reason a number of herbs belonging to them are also used to repel forces of evil.[34]

Table 5 gives a breakdown of all the principal *orixás* who control herbs that may be used for fumigation. It will be observed that Yemanjá stands out among all the others as being the *orixá* who controls or shares control of most of the herbs capable of being used to attract and repel, and the three *orixás* directly behind her are all feminine. The majority of herbs that may be used for fumigation therefore come under the control of feminine *orixás*. The powers of the herbs to attract good or repel evil are fairly evenly distributed, with the emphasis slightly more on the side of attracting than of repelling. The remaining *orixás* are all masculine, Oxalá still showing an emphasis on the ability to attract while Oxossi is equally powerful in both functions. Ogun and Omolú, however, show a definite movement away from the ability to attract in favour of the ability to repel.

Fumigatory rituals fall into two distinct categories. Either fumigation takes place as a preventive measure or it forms part of a definite curing ritual.

It is common in Bahia to fumigate the house every Saturday at 6 p.m. as a preventive measure to keep away any undesirable forces that may disrupt the harmony within (C.2, I.2, I.3, S.2).[35] In this case, the ingredients used would be both to attract good and repel evil, and they would all be included in the censer at the same time. Usually five or seven ingredients are employed, at least one of which must be known to be power-

Table 5. Numbers of herbs used in fumigation under the influence of each *orixá*.

	Herbs used in Fumigation		
Orixá	(*a*) *to attract*	(*b*) *to repel*	*Total*
Yemanjá	8	6	14
Oxun	4	4	8
Yansan	4	4	8
Naná	4	3	7
Oxalá	4	2	6
Oxossi	3	3	6
Ogun	1	4	5
Omolú	1	4	5

ful in repelling evil, the majority of the substances being sweet-smelling. Two very common mixtures used a lot in Cachoeira and sold already mixed in the market were (a) *alecrim*, *alfazema*, *tirateima*, *vencetudo*, incense; (b) *alecrim*, *alfazema*, *açafrão*, incense, storax, garlic straw, sugar. This is similar to the Portuguese custom of fumigating the house with *alecrim*, *arruda*, piassaba, powdered incense and rock salt all together, while crossing from one corner to another in each of the rooms.[36] In Brazil, however, the person fumigating must start at the back door and work his way through all the rooms of the house to the front door, when all the contents of the censer are thrown into the street (C.2 and *passim*).

However, if the ritual is being conducted for the specific purpose of ridding a patient of an evil force that is making him ill, or ridding his house of a similar force that is bringing disaster and misfortune to himself and his family, then the ritual must be divided up into two parts. It is considered of primary importance first to get rid of the evil causing the indisposition in question, and only after that to attract forces of good, because if a good force is attracted to and sealed in a place where an evil force reigns, the evil force may never be able to leave. The fumigation that forms part of a *sacudida* ritual consists, first, of burning powdered coffee and garlic straw, for example, followed by sugar and lavender or some other suitable substance. The censer is usually passed all round the patient, and particularly beneath each armpit. If the house is being fumigated, the person fumigating starts at the back door with ingredients that repel and throws all the contents of the censer through the front door into the street. The censer is then recharged with live coals and ingredients to attract good, and the person fumigating works from the open front door to the back door, which remains shut (I.2, C.2).

Fumigatory rituals are often accompanied by prayers and chants which find their origin mainly in Portugal. Valle gives the following from north Portugal, which is said while fumigating a house:

Just as Our Lady fumigated her beloved Son that he might smell sweet, so do I fumigate this house/person that all the evil inside might go away;[37]

and Leite de Vasconcellos quotes the following variation to cure a child:

Just as Our Lady fumigated her beloved Son that he might smell sweet, so do I fumigate you that the evil might leave you.[38]

In Itaparica, a similar prayer is sung to music:

1 Our Lady incensed her altar that her blessed Son might smell sweet. Incense, Our Lady, incense so that health and peace might enter [or] that her blessed Son might smell sweet. [I.2]

The origin of the words of this prayer is clearly Portuguese, though it is sometimes chanted in such a way as to appear more closely linked to the African *Candomblé* ceremonies. This is also the case with the following chants, in which one line is repeated over and over again with little melodic variation in characteristic African fashion:

2 Incense censer my grandfather's home. [I.2]

3 I have now fumigated (*bis*), O my Lady, [or] I am praising, I have now fumigated. [I.2]

It is very common in Brazil during spoken prayers which accompany fumigation to associate the ingredients in the censer with what one is trying to achieve by means of repeated similes, but this is usually the case only when fumigating to attract good. For example:

4 Just as this sugar is sweet, I before my enemies will sweeten. Just as this lavender smells sweet, I before them will smell sweet. With the power of God and the Virgin Mary. Amen. [I.2 and *passim*]

CHAPTER VII

RITUAL BATHS

The idea that ritual pollution can be removed by water is widespread and was certainly common to the three principal cultures that came together in Brazil. Water was considered to be akin to fire in that it was not only a purifier that could wash away all forms of uncleanness, but also a fertilizing agent that had the essential quality of being able to accomplish a transformation from one state to another. At the very basis of purification is the notion of fertility, because purification implies that some form of transformation is taking place:

The phenomenon of birth carries with it the ideas of the ceremonially unclean; hence the numerous precautions and taboos to be observed until the mother's *Churching*, that is, her first appearance at church. Under the same trend of ideas both mother and child are believed to be particularly exposed to the attack of demons; hence the precaution of having a burning candle by the bedside, fire being a well-known *apotropaion* ... The practice of putting new-born children on the fire, ... and the corresponding rite in which water is credited with having the beneficent effects attributed to fire in the previous one ... are but other forms taken on by the same set of primitive notions ...

Nor can one accept as the only possible one the usual interpretation of the baptismal rite as signifying a ceremonial cleaning. The idea of purification no doubt existed in fairly remote times. Yet equally old is the conception of water as the fertilizing element ... [Krappe 1930 1st ed 1962:222–3, 274).

The custom of washing the new-born among the Tupi tribes is based upon the same idea as baptism in the early Christian Church in that the new-born child is considered to be ceremonially unclean and must be purified in order to survive. A Tupinambá woman out of preference gave birth to her child close to water, usually on the banks of a river,[1] and as soon as the child was born, her husband washed it well and then proceeded with other rituals connected with protecting the child from evil or ensuring his future potential as a hunter.[2] A similar ritual is performed today among the Guayaki[3] and the Nambicuara.[4] Water in this instance transforms the child, taking it out of the state of impurity that accompanied the birth to a sacred state which ensures its ability to develop its relationships with the gods. The ritual bath not only forms part of every ritual undertaken during the major stages of a person's life (birth, puberty, initiation, marriage, etc.), but is taken on a day-to-day basis among many different tribes, and tribe members may take between seven and ten a day.[5]

The Pataxó Indians, who live in a FUNAI[6] reserve in the south of the state of Bahia, make a point of having a ritual bath before eating food and directly after entering a friend's house (P.1), and Karsten mentions how the Jibaro warrior must be ceremonially washed on his return from battle.[7] Such examples of ritual bathing among the Indian population of Brazil are legion, and the custom is clearly based on the notion that the bather achieves an exceptional state of purity which must be maintained by taking other baths periodically. Similar ideas concerning ritual purity are found elsewhere, too. Harper isolates three main stages in Havik Brahmin pollution rules whereby the middle stage is the normal every-day position and the highest and lowest stages mark the pure and impure states respectively. The highest position of purity can only be achieved by a rite of bathing, and it is only when in this position that the Brahmin can adequately worship his gods.[8]

This is also the case in the African religions of Brazil, where no ritual act, however small, can be undertaken without the parties concerned having bathed themselves shortly beforehand. The Africans undoubtedly took a lot of their ideas concerning bathing from Islam and brought these with them to Brazil.[9] Traditionally, cult houses should have a stream or river running through the land adjoining the house, and the water should be clean enough to be able to be used for all rituals during the year. *Filhas de santo* bathe themselves in the stream every morning, and water drawn from the stream goes into the clay pots representing the *orixás* in the *pejí* (sanctuary in the cult house) and forms the basis of the mixture in which the stones (known as *otá*) belonging to each *orixá*, and the beads belonging to the faithful of the cult, are washed.[10] Contact with the water heightens the person's and the object's sacred character and raises them to a higher spiritual plane.

Washing therefore has nothing to do with the removal of physical dirt—indeed, a ritual bath in Brazil usually consists of a tin of water simply tipped over the head—but it does remove all forms of pollution, which is essential before entering into contact with the gods.[11]Andrade points out how the adjective *sujo* (dirty) is a euphemism for the devil in

Portugal and Brazil, and quotes two quatrains that link the presence of the devil with ritual uncleanness, and washing with purification:

Flee enemies, back Satan! If the flesh were clean you would not do me evil. Amen.

Lady Sant'Ana you are our refuge! We are going to bathe to be rid of dirt.[12]

Pollution in Brazil is not as complex a matter as it can be in other societies,[13] a person being considered *de corpo sujo* (dirty of body) after either sexual intercourse or menstruation (I.2 and *passim*). Sometimes merely being in, or sleeping in, the same room as a member of the opposite sex can be considered ritually polluting, but this is not common (C.5).

In any ritual act, however small, the person concerned and all the onlookers must be *de corpo limpo* (clean of body), and this means that a ritual bath must have been taken shortly before the act. Hence a bath taken in the morning is not considered sufficiently purifying if one is to attend a ritual in the late afternoon, and there are often officials at the door of *Candomblé* rituals or spirit sessions who are watchful for signs that all members of the congregation have recently washed (I.7, C.2, C.8.). On one occasion in Itaparica a man was turned away at the door of a house where a spirit session was due to take place because his hair was not wet, and this implied to the officials present that he had not had a bath shortly before coming (I.7).

Care should be taken not to touch amulets when the body is impure, and *filhas de santo* hang up their beads before menstruation so as to ensure that they will not touch them by mistake when menstruating. Any object that should only be touched when the body is ritually pure immediately loses its power if touched when the body is unclean. If such defilement takes place deliberately, the person's *orixá* may punish the *filho/filha de santo* by forcing him or her, when possessed, to practise self-flagellation or to sleep on a bed of nettles. Leaves may not, under any circumstances, be picked when the picker is in an impure state, because they immediately lose their power, and it is believed in certain cases that grave damage can be done to the plant or tree. The *acoco* tree, for example, will wither and die if touched by someone who is ritually unclean (C.1, C.5).

The idea in many cultures that dealings with the sacred may only be undertaken by one person who is usually unmarried stems from the belief that sexual intercourse defiles. His or her chastity is the link between the world of men and the world of the gods. Moreover, the virginity of the priest is attributed power because his virginity sets him aside from other men and imparts to him the means of persuading the gods to do the will of man.[14] Celibacy among *Candomblé* priests is rare nowadays, but the Malé cult still observes it in its traditional houses (C.10), and it is a curious fact that many married *pais* or *mães de santo* no longer cohabit with their marriage partners through being legally separated.

The purificatory influence of pure water extends into the area of curing in that it can serve to remove evil influences from the body.[15] Lucas (1963:303–4) mentions how a bath on the night of the feast of St John removes all evil from the body, and that a childless couple should bathe naked for fertility; while in Brazil it is certainly common during spirit sessions for the president to sprinkle water over any patients present and to wash their faces with the water in the *copo de vidência*.[16]

Ritual bathing, however, becomes considerably more complex with the addition of different herbs and other substances. The possible combinations of herbs appear to be infinite, and in many cases it is the *orixá* of the *curandeiro* in question who dictates which specific herbs should be employed for each individual patient. The vast majority of herbs listed in Appendix One may be used for some kind of ritual bath, so the *curandeiro*'s knowledge of plant lore must be considerable and his fame as a *curandeiro* tends to be measured in terms of the extent of his skill in such matters. One informant in Cachoeira (C.1), who had been a *pai de santo* for twenty-eight years, admitted *eu ainda aprendo* ('I am still learning'), and this sums up the general attitude towards the use of herbs in baths. Their power is considered to be limitless provided it is harnessed in the correct way. One herb used by itself in a bath may be of little use, but combined with other herbs may take on enormous importance. It is futile to try to record the different combinations, because each individual's requirement is looked upon as being a special case that calls for specific combinations of herbs. A *curandeiro* does not prescribe for a particular illness; rather he prescribes for the individual who is ill. Parrinder (1969:157) records an identical viewpoint in Africa:

A young Agni woman when asked what leaves she used for treatment, said she did not know. But when she was in a trance, she plunged into the forest and plucked unthinkingly those leaves that came to hand. When we asked her if all sicknesses of the same type did not require the same treatment, she replied that no two sicknesses were alike, but that they depended on the people who are sick.

Curandeiros are under normal circumstances loath to part with their knowledge, and this is not based so much on a fear that their knowledge may at some future date be used against them as on the notion that herbs may lose their power if too many people who are not going to use them for the purpose for which they were created learn too much about them. There is a wide aura of mystery surrounding certain key herbs (such as *acoco*), which informants are unwilling to clarify.

Herbal baths come under the generic name of *banhos de cheiro* (perfumed baths), and as in the case of fumigators, there are basically two different types: one to repel forces of evil and the other to attract forces of good. Their functions, however, do go somewhat deeper than this, depending on the seriousness of the indisposition being cured.

Baths that are supposed to repel are called *banhos de descarga* or *discarrego*,[17] implying that their function is to unload and dispense with something weighing heavily on the patient. Herbs used in these baths are usually crushed in the bare hands and left to stand for a few moments in water. Then the whole mixture is tipped over the head. The patient, however, should not under any circumstances wipe himself dry or attempt to remove any of the leaves or twigs left sticking to his body or in his hair (I.2 and *passim*). The importance of leaving the *banho* to dry itself on the body has been noted elsewhere,[18] and seems to be based on the notion that the mixture should be allowed to soak in and thoroughly permeate the skin with its own particular perfume. One informant, C.5, suggested that the herbs, once combined in a *banho*, took on a particular cosmic power which it was above man's station to touch; hence it should be allowed to dry of its own accord.

The *orixás* that control the principal herbs used in *descarga* baths are shown in Table 6. Again, those *orixás* associated with physical strength (Yansan, Ogun) or the primeval powers of oceans and rivers (Yemanjá, Oxun) feature high on the list, together with Omolú, the smallpox god, who frightens away all evil with the threat of death.

The type of bath designed to attract good is called a *banho de desenvolvimento* (development bath), and as its name implies, it is supposed primarily to develop and refresh the mind. It is taken usually as a form of tonic, and herbs particularly favoured are those that have stood on the

Table 6. Number of herbs used in *descarga* baths under each *orixá*.

Orixá	*Number of Herbs Controlled*
Omolú	15
Yemanjá	14
Yansan	14
Oxun	13
Ogun	13
Naná	7
Oxossi	5
Exú	5
Oxalá	3

table during a spirit session and have therefore been close to the spirits as they manifested themselves. Flowers are also commonly employed in *desenvolvimento* baths, especially *angélica*, also called *flor de capela* (chapel flower). The leaves or flowers are put into a pan of water, which is brought to the boil and then immediately taken off the heat. As in the case of a *banho de descarga*, the entire contents are then tipped over the head when sufficiently cool and the body must not be wiped dry (I.2 and *passim*). Some *curandeiros* stipulate that a warm bath, known as *banho cozido* (cooked bath), should not be tipped over the head but only from the neck downwards, while raw baths should always be poured first over the head (C.1, C.2).[19] The *banho de desenvolvimento* may be taken by itself at any time during the day, but the *banho de descarga* is usually immediately followed either by fumigation with substances to attract good, or by a *banho de desenvolvimento*.[20] This may be connected with the notion that any evil force must be dispensed with before endeavouring to attract a good force, as we have already observed in the case of fumigation. However, it may also be linked to the fact that one bath (*descarga*) is raw, and the other (*desenvolvimento*) is cooked, and for this reason the one should follow the other. Harper has pointed out how Havik Brahmins make a distinction between cooked and raw food as carriers of pollution. Cooked food may pass on pollution while raw food will not.[21] I feel there may be a similarity here with the two types of bath in Brazil in that the raw bath always precedes the cooked one. The raw bath purifies and annihilates any force that may become malignant, while the cooked bath fortifies the good forces that remain.

Table 7 shows the *orixás* that control the principal herbs employed for *banhos de desenvolvimento*. It will be observed that Omolú now no longer

Table 7. Number of herbs used in *desenvolvimento* baths under each *orixá*.

Orixá	*Number of Herbs Controlled*
Oxun	14
Yemanjá	14
Yansan	11
Ogun	10
Naná	8
Omolú	6
Oxossi	5
Oxalá	5
Exú	4

plays a major role, while Ogun features among the first four principal *orixás*. One of the principal characteristics of the *banho de desenvolvimento* is development and expansion of the spirit, and one of Ogun's functions is to *abrir caminhos*[22] ('open the ways') with his sword in the sense of clearing away difficulties and establishing a smooth path to follow.

Oxun, Yemanjá and Yansan feature high on both lists because they have a double-sided nature already noted above[23] whereby they are equally able to play a role involving physical force and to show the gentleness more normally associated with the female sex.

Desenvolvimento baths as here described are usually taken at the patient's discretion, and he will acquire his herbs either growing wild or at a herb stall in a market. *Descarga* baths, however, are usually, but not always, prescribed by *curandeiros*, who may in some cases consult their personal *orixás*.

There are also, as in the case of fumigators, large numbers of marketed varieties of *banhos* which are readily available in market stalls and appear to enjoy the same sales turnover as marketed fumigators. In fact they are similar to marketed fumigators in every way, and display the same characteristic titles and woodcuts on the packets. They either consist of leaves that are finely crushed (and thereby rendered unrecognizable) or they are sold in liquid form in bottles. The packet usually advises the patient to say a prayer such as the Hail Mary or Our Father on taking the bath, though one variety found in Bahia but manufactured in Rio de Janeiro suggested accompanying the bath with the following prayer in Latin. It is transcribed complete with errors.

Ore: Accipiati quaesemuus Domine Deus noster, bene, dictionem tuam creatura tua ista, qua corpore, salvetur, et mente comgruam-que tibi exbibiat servitutem a tue tuae propiationins beneficiasemper—in—veniat Per Christur. Amem.

Curandeiros use two other types of bath—both of them extensions of the *descarga* and *desenvolvimento* baths studied so far—which are of prime importance in curing particularly serious or complex cases. These are called *abó* and *amasi.*[24] In traditional houses, they form part of every major ritual, especially those connected with initiation and the advancement of the initiate up the ladder of the priestly hierarchy. The *iaô* (initiate) must have an *abó* bath every day and drink some of the mixture before pouring it over her head. The mixture is also splashed on the ground over which the initiate walks, so as to purify it and ward off all danger.[25] *Abó* baths are taken by participants in *obi* and *bori* ceremonies which are rituals that allow the person involved to renew his faith and devotion to his *orixá* at a somewhat higher level than initiation.[26] Often the *abó* bath, whenever taken, is followed by an *amasi.* It is true that in *Candomblé de caboclo* cult houses the *abó* and *amasi* baths are also employed at certain stages of normal everyday ritual, but they have also come to be used by *curandeiros* to cure serious illnesses that will not respond to simpler treatment (e.g. baths of a less complex nature discussed above). In traditional cult houses they mark a turning-point during particular rituals, and in the same way they serve to mark a turning-point in the treatment of disease.

The components of the *abó* are very secret, and members of the priestly hierarchy of traditional cult houses would never divulge such information. Ramos describes it as *um banho de folhas aromáticas, que só os pais e mães de santo conhecem*[27] ('a bath of aromatic leaves, known only by *pais* and *mães de santo*'), and Câmara Cascudo says it is *um banho aromático cujas ervas só são conhecidas pelo Pai ou Mãe-de-Santo*[28] ('an aromatic bath the constituent herbs of which are only known by a *pai* or *mãe de santo*'). *Candomblé de caboclo* informants show the same resistance when asked to detail the components of the *abó*, but in certain houses in Cachoeira and Itaparica, the following recipes for an *abó* bath were obtained:

A *alecrim*
aroeira
folha da Costa

espada de Ogun
macaça
grated *obi* nut
river/rain water
honey
blood of sacrificial animal
[C.1]

B *acoco*
aroeira
betis branco
cajá
coerana
espada de Ogun
narciso branco
São Gonçalinho
grated *obi* nut
river/rain water
blood of sacrificial animal
[C.8]

C *alecrim*
aluman
angélica
aroeira
arruda
catinga de porco
catinga de crioula
coerana
espada de Ogun
espada de Oxossi
espada de Yansan
guiné
lança de Oxalá
pinhão roxo
tapete de Oxalá
vassourinha de Nossa Senhora
garlic straw

grated *obi* nut
rock salt
river/rain water
blood of sacrificial animal
[C.6]

D *aroeira*
capianga
espinho cheiroso
guiné
muricí
São Gonçalinho
tirateima
vencetudo
blood of sacrificial animal
river/rain water
[I.2]

All four informants agreed that the number of leaves that enter the *abó* should be five, nine, twelve or twenty-one. The leaves should ideally all be different, but quantities may be made up by using more than one sample of one leaf. All leaves that go into the *abó* must be picked very early in the morning, preferably between 3 and 4 a.m. In this case, normal taboos with regard to hours of picking are waived when appropriate. The animal concerned in the sacrifice is normally the animal dedicated to the principal *orixá* presiding over the cult house in question. The mixture is made up in a jar with a lid, and this is then either buried or suspended at a height of about six feet against the trunk of one of the following trees: *dendê*, *jaqueira* or *cajá*. The mixture is then left for a period of at least twelve days, during which it putrifies, though it is best to keep it as long as possible. The best *abó* mixtures are those made at the beginning of the year and used whenever required, the mixture being topped up from time to time whenever necessary.[29] The *abó* bath, after a while, takes on an extremely pungent, rotten smell, but it is taboo at all times to refer to its unpleasant odour with any word other than *cheiro*, which implies a sweet smell. If a word like *feder* (to stink) is used, the *abó* will have a purely maleficent effect.

It will be noted that all four informants give different herbs that often do not coincide with those in the other recipes, *aroeira* being the only one included in all of them. I.2 concluded her list by saying that *todas as ervas fortes* ('all the strong herbs') could be included if considered necessary. Each recipe, however, contains ingredients that between them give a very fair representation of all the *orixás*, and the addition of blood and the *obi* nut raise the level of the *abó* beyond that of other types of *banho* we have already examined. Blood is the all-powerful ingredient, and animals are sacrificed throughout the year because the shedding of their blood provides essential energy and food for the *orixás*,[30] while the *obi* nut is attributed great powers and used in most important rituals, including divination.[31] The *abó* bath therefore provides a strong link with the world of the gods, and many people, on taking it, fall into a trance, while it is also common for the mere smell of the liquid to induce a trance state (I.2 and *passim*).[32] It is this proximity to the power of the spirit world that can expel the most maleficent spirits believed to be the cause of illness.

The *abó* bath must, under all circumstances, be taken raw, because *o que vive dá vida* ('what is alive gives life') (C.1.). The body must not be wiped dry, but as in the case of other *banhos*, allowed to dry itself. In certain cases, all the remnants of the herbs used that fall to the floor must be collected, dried out and then burned (I.4, C.5, C.6).

The *amasi* bath, when used as a means of curing, often follows the *abó* directly. It has a complementary function in relation to the *abó*, whose effect is not complete without the final 'seal' of the *amasi*. Whereas the *abó* is of fixed ingredients, the herbs that go into the *amasi* often vary in accordance with the preferences of each *orixá*. Hence a person belonging to an *orixá* will take an *amasi* made up of herbs that come under the particular control of his *orixá*. The individual composition of the *amasi* with respect to the patient's *orixá* finds its origin in traditional houses. Bastide, with reference to the *amasi* in the Nagô cult, calls it *um banho em cuja composição entram folhas especiais pertencentes ao respectivo Orixá*[33] ('a bath in the composition of which enter special leaves belonging to the respective *orixá*'). Binon Cossard, however, implies that the *amasi* (in the Angola cult) is made up strictly in accordance with the individual's requirements, and mentions an *amasi* of herbs chosen specifically to keep away the *egun*.[34]

However, it would appear that, certainly in the case of *Candomblé de caboclo*, there is a fixed number of herbs and other ingredients that must form the base of the *amasi* to which other herbs, depending on the case in question, are added. Two lists of stock herbs were obtained as follows:

E *bonina*
cajá
manjericão
sangolovo
grated *obi* nut
blood of sacrificial animal
[C.1]

F *acoco*
aroeira
betis branco
cajá
narciso branco
São Gonçalinho
blood of sacrificial animal
[C.8]

As in the case of the *abó* bath, the herbs included in both the recipes for *amasi* are all different, with the exception of *cajá*, which features in both recipes.

The main difference between the *abó* and the *amasi* is that the *amasi* is not allowed to putrify, and hence its smell is a pleasant one. It is made by crushing the different leaves in water and then allowing the mixture to stand for at least two to three hours, and sometimes overnight. Like the *abó*, it is always taken raw and tipped over the head, and again, the body should not be wiped dry.

CHAPTER VIII

PEMBA (RITUAL POWDER)

Pemba is a powder that is used during many *Candomblé* rituals and also as a means of curing. The importance of it in ritual is accounted for in a myth:

Even after marrying Oshun, Shango continued going to feasts by himself, having a good time and various adventures with women. Oshun complained about remaining at home alone and so they had a row . . . For this reason he locked her away in a tower in his palace. One day, Eshu Etameta, the owner of the crossroads, arrived at a crossroads in front of Shango's palace. He saw Oshun crying on the veranda and asked her the reason. She told him the story and he then went and told it to Orumila. Orumila prepared an *ishe* [a powder of magic leaves] and told Eshu to tell her to leave her window open. He then blew on the powder which went through the window and transformed Oshun into a dove. She flew back to her father's house where he transformed her back. This is the reason why Oshun does not eat doves.[1]

Bastide mentions the same magical powder (. . . *pó talismã, o Ixê* . . .) that is rubbed into tattoo marks during the process of initiation.[2] The words *ishe* and *ixê* are clearly linked with *exé**, which was given to me in Itaparica by I.2 as an alternative way of referring to *pemba*.

As in the case of fumigators and baths, there are marketed varieties of *pemba* as well as those that can be prepared in the home. The marketed varieties fall into two distinct categories in that they can be either solid or powdered. An elemental analysis of the solid variety revealed that it is made up mainly of kaolin with 0.21 per cent carbon and 1.94 per cent hydrogen.[3] Its consistency is the same as chalk, and originally it came in two shapes, one oval and the other circular. The oval shape is by far the most common, and although informants (C.5, C.10) speak of the existence of the circular type, I never came across an example. These shapes are called masculine and feminine respectively, but since the feminine shape is now no longer common, this distinction of sex is rarely made.[4] Solid *pemba* is also made in different colours corresponding to each *orixá*.

Solid *pemba* is used particularly in *Candomblé de caboclo* cult houses, but it is also being used more frequently nowadays in more traditional houses. Its principal function is to draw marks on the body, particularly during initiation, and during ceremonies such as the *bori*. In one *bori* ceremony performed by C.1 and witnessed in Cachoeira, solid white *pemba* was scraped with the sacrificial knife and the resulting powder made to fall first over the person's head, then over the whole body, and finally over the sheet on which the person was sitting. It was then used to draw lines on the soles and upper parts of the feet. Binon Cossard mentions its use during the ceremony that takes place after the death of one of the *filhas de santo* in which the *pai de santo* uses it to draw a vertical line on his forehead and cheeks, a horizontal line on his eyelids and a cross on the palms of his hands.[5]

Its main use, however, in *Candomblé de caboclo* cult houses, is for curing, where it is used like chalk to draw certain cabbalistic signs on the floor inside which the curer or the patient stands while the ritual is being performed.[6] Examples of these signs and rituals are given below in Chapter XI.

The notion of drawing some cabbalistic sign on the floor as an aid to the priest's power is a borrowing from Europe,[7] and such signs now play an extremely important role in *Umbanda* and *Macumba*, in the south of Brazil, particularly Rio de Janeiro and São Paulo. Each *santo* or spirit is allocated his or her sign, and the tracing of such a sign on the floor (*ponto riscado*) is believed to attract the spirit into the presence of the priest and his followers (R.1).[8] The fact that solid *pemba* should be used to draw such signs may be based on the recommendations in early texts that only substances that have undergone rigorous ritual preparation are efficacious for any esoteric practice. Most grimoires draw attention to the enormous importance attached to the ritual preparation of substances and tools that must take place before any esoteric ceremony as described in the grimoire is undertaken. The *Grimoire of Pope Honorius* underlines the necessity of using coal and 'consecrated chalk' to draw the cabbalistic circle in which the sorcerer stands,[9] and it is not unlikely that such detailed instructions as these in early texts provide the origin of the use of solid *pemba* for the drawing of similar signs in Brazil.

The other type of marketed *pemba* is always in powdered form, and is sold in small packets measuring on average $1\frac{1}{2}'' \times \frac{3}{4}'' \times \frac{1}{4}''$. Each packet states the purpose for which the contents should be used in the title: e.g. *Domínio* (Dominion): *Chama Dinheiro* ('money caller'); *Vencedora de Batalha* ('battle winner'); *Amarra marido* ('husband bringer'); *Pega Homem* ('man getter'); *Pega Mulher* ('wife getter'); *Amansa Sogra* ('mother-in-law sweetener'). Some packets just bear the names of certain herbs that have supposedly gone towards their manufacture: e.g. *Vence Tudo* ('overcome everything'); *Abre Caminhos* ('open the ways'). However, analysis of such *pembas* revealed that their herbal content was minimal and that they were made up principally of kaolin with 0.67 per cent carbon and 0.14 per cent nitrogen.

A number of the packets are decorated with woodcuts, e.g. a dancing couple on *Pega Homem*, an angel on *Pó da Felicidade* ('happiness powder',) but some of them are very curious and bear little relation to the function of the *pemba* in question. *Amansa Sogra*, for example, displays a picture of what appears to be a prostitute, while *Pó de Separação* ('separation powder') shows a wise owl with a mortar-board on its head.

Powdered forms of marketed *pemba* differ only very slightly in colour, the predominant colour being white. They also all have the same basic smell, which is very similar to that of cheap talcum powder. In fact, they are most commonly used as talcum powder, the idea being that the function inherent in the title will be sympathetically passed on to the wearer. Some varieties, however, require to come into physical contact with two or more people. Hence a man wanting to attract a woman must put some *Pega Mulher* on his hands and then endeavour to touch the woman he is interested in. A person wanting to increase his circle of friends does likewise with *Amizade* (Friendship), and so on (C.8).

Waite (1911:301) mentions a similar idea found in the *Book of True Black Magic*, which advises the sorcerer who wants to conjure up a certain person at a given moment into his presence that '. . . a powder must be made and cast upon the person, or given them with their meat or drink'. Instructions given by the *Grand Grimoire* to make people appear naked and dance in one's presence involve the collection of certain herbs at midnight on the eve of the feast of St John. These herbs are pounded into a powder, which must then be sprinkled in the air of the room where the desired people are present.[10]

Marketed varieties of *pemba* of both forms all come from Rio de Janeiro, São Paulo or Porto Alegre, despite assurances on the packet that they are *Africano Legítimo* (Legitimate African), imported especially from Africa. The instruction leaflet for solid *pemba* shows pictures of *pemba* being made in a large cauldron by a number of Africans and another picture of the finished product being delivered to the market in Lagos, *Africa do Sul* (South Africa) (*sic*), and it ends with the following warning:

Buying a false *pemba* involves, besides losing your money, running the risk of attracting evil influences on using it. Care! Great care! The only exporter for the entire world is Ali-Bem-Itah of the Umbanda Tribe, a direct descendent of Soba L-U-Thab.

On the packet, however, is stated quite clearly:

Specially made by the Livraria e Flora Olimpia Ltda.—Porto Alegre—Rio Grande do Sul.

The packet also gives the number of the Brazilian patent. The powdered *pemba* called *Separação* says on one side that it is *Legítimo Africano*, and on the other *E.E.U.U.* (the accepted Brazilian abbreviation for Estados Unidos—United States).

Generally, marketed *pemba* of the powdered variety is used by private individuals without previous recommendation from higher authority, but it is also used a great deal by certain *Candomblé de caboclo* priests in curing rituals. Home-made *pemba*, however, is always considered to be much superior to the marketed varieties in that all the ingredients are known and the quantities of each substance can be adjusted to suit the maker's wishes. To make *pemba* in the home, however, requires painstaking work on the part of the *pai* or *mãe de santo*, who must devote long hours to reducing the ingredients to as fine a powder as the average talcum. This is one reason why marketed *pembas* are so popular and looked upon with considerably less suspicion than marketed fumigators or baths, the main reason perhaps being that the majority of marketed *pembas*, especially those of the solid varieties, are believed to have come direct from Africa. It is significant in this respect that a number of recipes for home-made *pemba* include marketed white *pemba* of the solid variety among the ingredients.

Pemba that is made in the home is called *pemba preparada* to distinguish it from marketed varieties. Its main ingredients are herbs and seeds, but sometimes sugar, myrrh, incense and solid white marketed *pemba* are also included. Complete individual recipes are jealously guarded since each person considers his recipe to be the most powerful and is very loath to part with any information concerning it. I was able, however, to collect the following three:

1 solid white *pemba* (marketed)
sugar

angélica do sertão
capianga
dandá
murici
poejo
quitoco
tira teima
vencetudo
[I.2]

2 *acoco*
água de Levante
dandá
(preferably picked on the first Friday of Lent)
[C.5]

3 incense
myrrh
white talcum powder/solid *pemba*
alfazema
dandá
noz moscada
cinnamon
1 clove
[C.2]

The herbs employed must be dried in the sun, though they may be dried artificially (as in an oven) if the *pemba* is required urgently.[11] When dry, all the ingredients must be crushed together in a mortar and passed repeatedly through a muslin cloth in order to acquire a fine powder.

Sometimes the white *pemba* (which belongs to Oxalá) can be exchanged for other solid *pembas* of different colours that belong to different *orixás*, depending on the *orixá* who happens to hold the most sway over the person in question. This is the only instance in the case of *pemba* where feelings for an individual's *orixá* may be taken into consideration, the normal course being to distribute precisely the same *pemba* to anyone in need of it.

The principal herbs among those in Appendix One that may be used for the manufacture of *pemba preparada* show a fairly even spread among all the *orixás*, as Table 8 shows, with emphasis on Yemanjá and Oxun.

Table 8. Number of herbs used to make *pemba preparada* under each *orixá*.

Orixá	*Number of Herbs Controlled*
Yemanjá	7
Oxun	6
Ogun	4
Yansan	4
Oxossi	2
Omolú	2
Naná	2
Oxalá	1
Xangô	1

This is a reflection of the notion that *pemba* summons the assistance of all the gods at the same time, it being up to the individual concerned to increase the reliance on one particular *orixá* if he so desires by the addition of the relevant solid *pemba*.

During the manufacture of *pemba*, the person concerned must be ritually clean, otherwise it will turn out to have no power at all. It is also necessary to accompany all stages of its manufacture with prayers and incantations. The prayers are often of a spontaneous kind, and follow no rigid outlines, and they take the form of an invocation to the gods (who are either the *orixás* or the three different members of the Catholic Trinity) to impart some of their power to the *pemba* currently being made. Two such prayers are as follows:

1 With the forces of God and of all the *orixás*, with all the forces which God left in heaven, earth, sea and star, I ask you all that you make this *pemba* which I am preparing of benefit to me and to all who may make use of it. [I.2]

2 *Pemba*, I prepare you in the name of the Father, the Son and the Holy Ghost to do good. [C.6]

The incantations accompanying the manufacture of *pemba* should number at least three (according to I.2), and should be repeated over and over again, together with the prayer, until the *pemba* is complete. Incantations are either of the type that are specifically designed to be used with *pemba*, or they are borrowed from another ritual called *ingolosi*. The former varieties are transcribed below. The original language is a mixture of Portuguese (here given in translation) and a very corrupt and unidentifiable form of the language usually employed in traditional *Angola* cult houses:

3 O *pemba*, *pemba de lei*,[12] *pemba*. [I.2]

4 O *pemba*, come here samba, Angola samba. O *pemba*, send *pemba*.

5 *Pemba* was *de lei*, *pembé*, *pemba*.

Ingolosi (known in Portuguese as *rezas* = prayers) is the name given to a session of formal sung prayer that takes place on specific days of the week in traditional cult houses in the presence of all the members of the priestly hierarchy and *filhas de santo* who live in the cult house. It is rather akin to the office said daily by Catholic priests and nuns.[13] The incantations sung are extremely secret, and only one informant [I.2] was prepared to let me have a sample of those she knew.[14] These are transcribed here, and at least three of them may be sung during the preparation of *pemba*:

6 I put my knee on the ground asking for the love of God, Oxalá, to have patience, O Father, and mercy for this *orixá*.

The incantation is then repeated several times, substituting in the place of Oxalá the names of different *orixás*.

7 Help me my Mother, the Lady of the deep river. Help me my Mother, for the sake of the Saviour of the world.

8 Your mercy is limitless. Omolú asked for mercy in the cult house.

This incantation is also repeated several times, substituting in the place of Omolú the names of different *orixás*.

9 O what mercy from all the *orixás*.

10 Long live the rosary of the Virgin Mary. God came down from heaven, long may it live.

11 Get up, come and play, girl, at the table of the Father, girl, take the blessing of the most elderly, girl, at the table of the Father, girl, take the blessing of the brothers, girl.

The resulting *pemba* is widely used, not only as an important part of most curing rituals, but also in isolation. It is supposed to help one *se desenvolver*—that is, like the *desenvolvimento* bath it serves as a tonic—but its usual function is to protect the wearer from disease and all forms of the evil eye. It is common to take it by itself with hot water as a ritual bath, and directly afterwards to dust it all over the body. Many *pais* and *mães de santo* include it as an important ingredient inside amulets (particularly *breves* or *patuás*: see below, page 81).[15] It is also used a great deal after fumigating the house. A small heap is placed on the open palm of the right hand, and it is then blown into every room to the accompaniment of three or more of the incantations given above (I.2).

Pemba de Exú (*pemba* of Exú) or *pemba preta* (black *pemba*) refers to a variety of *pemba* that may only be used for evil purposes. Again there are two types, one marketed (always of the solid variety) and the other home made. An analysis of black-marketed *pemba* revealed that it was made up mainly of kaolin with 5 per cent carbon and 2 per cent hydrogen, and a minimal quantity of organic material.

The use of the home-made variety is extremely widespread, and many ills and misfortunes are attributed to it. During preparation it is treated with a great deal of care and respect, since it is believed to be one of the most powerful ways of inflicting harm on others, and a stray grain could react against the person preparing it. Everything to do with the manufacture of *pemba preta* must at all times remain outside the house. The pestle and mortar used to pound the ingredients into a powder, including the spoon used to transfer the ingredients into bottles, must only ever be used for *pemba preta*. Nothing that has touched it can be used for anything else, nor may anything that has been in contact with it be brought into the house. People who have used it must eliminate all traces of it from their hands by rubbing them with a freshly picked leaf, taking care to leave the leaf in the gutter or a drain (I.2, C.2, C.5, C.6). After this, on entering their houses, they must sprinkle sugar (left in advance at the front door) in every room, and then undertake the ritual known as *o despacho da porta*. This involves throwing the contents of a glass of water in three directions just outside the front door (I.2). It is a curious ritual that may be linked to the purifying power of water, though it is more likely to take the form of an offering of a drink to Exú, the guardian of all entrances, so that he will prevent any evil force coming into the house after the occupant has been using *pemba preta*. Offerings to Exú to prevent mishaps occurring are very common and are given before most rituals to ensure the smooth running of the ceremony. They are known as the *pade de Exú*,[16] translated into Portuguese as *despacho de Exú*, and this may be the main idea behind the ritual *o despacho da porta*.

Details concerning the manufacture of black *pemba* are kept very secret since each individual believes he has the all-powerful recipe and is extremely wary of passing it on to others out of a fear that it may ultimately be used against himself. Moreover, informants are often embarrassed when asked to expand on the details concerning back *pemba* since they feel that they might be giving the impression that they dabble too much in 'black', that is evil, ritual practices. They are, however, always very careful to point out how important it is for them to know the workings of 'black' practices so that they can operate against them for the good of their patients. Conversations concerning black *pemba* or 'black' ritual acts of any kind are always hurried, and informants do not like to expand too much. One informant, C.2, insisted on talking about black *pemba* outside in the yard and not in his house through fear that some evil might come of it.

Ingredients for *pemba preta* tend to include things that are normally associated with uncleanness (e.g. nicotine) and death (e.g. cemetery dirt), but it must also contain certain herbs, fruits and animals that come directly under the control of Exú, because Exú, when invoked in the correct way, can undertake acts of evil against other people.

Recipes I managed to collect are as follows:

A black-marketed *pemba* (solid)
pimenta da Costa
pimenta malagueta } (hot peppers of the chili type)
horse droppings
cansanção
corredeira
nettle
ash

salt
toad (dried then powdered)
cemetery dirt
[I.2]

B *corredeira*
louco branco
pimenta da Costa
pimenta malagueta
ants' nest earth
cemetery dirt
[C.2]

C toad
human bone
humming bird (black)
[C.5]

These are stored in alcohol until Holy Week, and then are toasted in a dish over a fire all at once. Then they are reduced to a fine powder with a pestle and mortar.

D toad dried and reduced to a fine powder

E *mangangá* wasp[17]
dragon fly
chameleon
bat
toad's skin
locust
liquid nicotine that accumulates in a pipe
dung beetle[18]
spider crab
scorpion
lizard
hair of black cat
hair of a vixen
dirt from the grave of a sorcerer

dust from a night club
seven *Urubú* feathers[19]
dust from seven crossroads
seven *pimentas da Costa*
one human bone
one live snake
[C.6]

All these ingredients are toasted in a new earthenware pot, which must afterwards be broken and included in the *pemba*.

F A certain lizard,[20] lays its egg inside the bark of *jasmin do Plário*. When the egg hatches the bark splits and the baby lizard emerges. The lizard, if grated during the months of May or June, can be used by itself as *pemba preta*. [C.1]

Recipes A, B and E contain peppers of different varieties. These, mainly because of the heat they produce in the mouth on being eaten, belong to Exú. Peppers must at all times be treated with a great deal of care because it is believed that, if they are bruised or fall to the ground inside the house, Exú will become angry and cause arguments and internal family disputes to break out.[21]

Plants and insects that sting are associated with Exú and hence are included among the ingredients. The mud-walls of the insects' nests are also included in this category.[22] Dragonflies (Recipe E) are most probably only included because in Portuguese they are known as *cavalos do cão* (horses of the dog, i.e. of the devil).[23] Sometimes it is sufficient for the animal simply to be black to qualify for inclusion among the ingredients (for example, Recipe C, black humming bird), but the *urubú*, which is also black, is most probably included mainly because it lives off carrion. The toad and the frog occur very commonly in European witchcraft,[24] and Pardal mentions the use of the toad in sorcery by Indians of the Tupi stock.[25]

In Recipe E it is important that all the insects/animals mentioned should be toasted alive over the fire together with all the other ingredients. The fire itself should be kindled with twigs from bushes and plants that come under the control of Exú, and the person preparing the *pemba* should take care to sit in such a way that the smoke from the fire does not blow over him, otherwise he may become contaminated.

Black *pemba* should be made on a Friday at midnight and preferably at a crossroads. Directly after its preparation, it should be bottled and buried for seven days before use. Incantations and prayers must also accompany the preparation of black *pemba*, the incantations being those normally sung during the *pade de Exú* at the commencement of a *Candomblé* festival.[26] I was able to obtain the following prayer said during the preparation of black *pemba*:

12 Black *pemba*, I toast you in the name of the Devil by the power of Satanás and Farrabás[27] and the prince Boizebú[28] and Maria Padrilha and all the family.[29] [C.6]

Prayers, usually of a spontaneous nature, stating the desired effects of the *pemba*, are generally said at the commencement of any evil ritual act. The following prayer, for example, was employed when it was desired to bring evil on a certain family:

13 Just as this black *pemba* has twenty-one ingredients, the twenty-one Exús of the twenty-one crossroads take over this house;[30] [C.6]

and accompanied by the action of blowing the *pemba* through the keyhole. Similar prayers would be said on placing *pemba* on the palm of the hand, as already described (page 66), and blowing it over objects or areas associated with the person on whom it was desired to bring misfortune.

The idea of blowing maleficent powder with the object of producing ruin dates back certainly as far as the witchcraft trials of the late sixteenth century in Europe, as the following passage from Rémy (1595 1st edn. 1930:67) shows:

Alexia Violaea bore witness that, after running here and there like the Bacchantes with her companions, she used to scatter in the air a fine powder given to her by the Demon for that purpose; and that from this were generated caterpillars, bruchuses, locusts, and such pests of the crops in such numbers that the fields on all sides were at once covered with them.

Apart from being blown in the air, *pemba* may also be used to write the name of an enemy on a piece of paper which is subsequently burned. It is also used as an essential ingredient in mixtures of specific components used in evil practices (C.2). This, too, has clear European antecedents, as may be seen in the Arcipreste de Hita's *Libro de Buen Amor* (440):

Toma de unas viejas, que se fasen erveras,
Andan de casa en casa e llámanse parteras;
Con polvos é afeytes é con alcoholeras,
Echan la moça en ojo é çiegan bien de veras.

(She takes into her service old women who parade as herbalists,
They go from house to house calling themselves midwives;
With powders, pomades and antimony,
They put the evil eye on the girl and render her totally blind).

In Brazil, black *pemba* may be sewn into a toad's mouth, together with the victim's name or photograph; the toad is then subjected to whatever treatment the sorcerer wishes his victim to undergo (C.2).

Sacrifices may be made to Exú for the specific purpose of his doing evil, at a crossroads, within the confines of a *ponto riscado* drawn with black *pemba* (C.2, C.5). All crossroads come under the control of Exú, but some are considered to be more propitious than others for sacrificial ends and it is common for a crossroads to be referred to as *uma encruzilhada boa que tem um Exú bom* ('a good crossroads that has a good Exú') (C.2).

CHAPTER IX

AMULETS

Amulets in Brazil may be worn as a means of protection in three areas: against the evil eye and the ill wind; against illnesses in particular or in general; against accidental and unforeseen occurrences. Most amulets, however, are manufactured and worn to protect the wearer against the perils of the evil eye and the ill wind, though these, as we shall see in the next chapter, are fairly elastic terms which can be stretched to include most other forms of indisposition. An amulet can be manufactured and worn for the specific purpose of guarding against a particular misfortune, but it is much more common for one amulet to be worn as a means of protection against general misfortune.

Amulets designed to give protection against general misfortune are generally considered less powerful than amulets consecrated for a specific purpose, though the efficacy of the latter is usually limited to the purpose stated. If the maker concentrates on the future owner's specific requirements while making the amulet, then that amulet will be rendered the more powerful an instrument in safeguarding its future owner (I.2 and *passim*).[1] One specific type of amulet may therefore be consecrated by different makers for different purposes. Hence a *figa*[2] may be worn to ensure easy delivery of a child. After the birth it may be discarded in favour of another *figa*, specially consecrated to make it more suited to the needs of a nursing mother and that would, for example, guarantee a ready flow of breast milk during the first weeks after the birth of the child.

The amulet in Brazil is usually worn around the wrist or the neck on a string or chain so that it is near the pulse or heart,[3] and its main function as a means of protection is rather akin to that of a lightning conductor. It attracts the force which, once attracted, is rendered completely harmless, and so the wearer of the amulet remains protected.[4] Sometimes the force of evil attracted into the amulet is so great that the amulet breaks, though informants stress that this is rare. There is, however, a reference to such a mishap actually happening to a *figa* in a Portuguese ballad:

Look at that devil of a woman!
The eyes that she put upon me!
I immediately began to tremble,
And then the *figa* broke.[5]

Traditionally, great importance was attached to the quality of the substance out of which amulets were made, mainly for the reason that poor-quality substances would not be able to withstand powerful forces of evil and the wearer might, as a result, be exposed to danger. Jet has always been considered a highly appropriate substance for the manufacture of amulets in Europe, and particularly in Spain and Portugal,[6] and it is much sought after today by Brazilian *curandeiros*. In the past, however, distinctions could be made between the varying qualities of jet to be found in the Iberian peninsula based on its ability or inability to withstand powerful forces. A document from the municipal archives of Santiago, dated 1581, praises jet found in Asturias while it condemns the jet from Monte Alban and Portugal, which shows a marked tendency to break:[7]

... in Monte Alban and in the Kingdom of Portugal there is a great deal of false jet, and being such, it is called dead and false, for it cannot withstand heat or wind; it rends and breaks on exposure to sun and wind and has not the strength of the fine Asturian jet, which comes from the principality of Asturias and which withstands wind and sun, unlike that of Monte Alban and of Portugal ...[8]

The same document goes on to describe how the use of jet was very strictly controlled by the authorities, who went to great pains only to allow high-quality jet to be employed because:

... if this were not done ... people would not know which was the fine variety or the dead one, and there could therefore be a great deal of fraud and deception practised on people and pilgrims who bought such jet, for it would soon break up.[9]

There is a large number of objects and signs which are used as amulets because of their specific shape, substance or smell: the *figa*, animal teeth/horns, cowrie shells, garlic, the pentangle, rings, herbs, nuts and seeds.

Perhaps the most common of them all is the *figa*. The *figa* is usually of the left hand, though I have seen it of the right hand on occasions. Some sources believe that the right-handed *figa* is more ancient than the left-handed one, but the left-handed *figa* is certainly the more common of the two nowadays.[10]

In Galicia, it is still common when a person meets a hunchback (believed to be a source of the evil eye) to make a *figa* with one of the hands and say:

Bread in the hand.
Bread in the basket.
Gee up donkey.
Take this away. [G.1]

Valle (1963:598–9) transcribes an identical rhyme from Portugal. The rhyme itself is mostly gibberish, but this in itself is considered a powerful way of repelling forces of evil, and it is rendered even more powerful with the addition of the *figa* gesture. Recitation of a ritual formula accompanied by the *figa* gesture when coming across an enemy has been recorded in north-east Brazil by Gomes (1951:190), the words in this instance being:

Dead man's *figa* to you . . .

Making the *figa* gesture with the hands and reciting such formulas, however, is not at all common now, it being considerably more usual simply to wear a carved *figa* round the neck or wrist. Street vendors usually either wear a *figa* or stand a large one up on their trays so as to protect their goods from the evil eye and ensure good sales throughout the day.[11]

The substances out of which a *figa* may be made vary enormously. Ideally, the strongest *figas* are made of jet, as already mentioned, but this is very rarely found in Brazil and never found for sale in markets. *Jacarandá* wood is extremely popular for the manufacture of *figas*, perhaps because it is often almost black in colour, very hard, and can bear a close resemblance to jet. Nowadays, more and more *figas* are found made of different coloured plastics or glass, the colours usually being those associated with the principal *orixás*. *Curandeiros*, however, spurn such materials and advise patients to buy or have made *figas* with *guiné* wood or *arruda*. Both these plants are widely used in Brazil for repelling the evil eye and for curing in general, and the leaves are among the most popular in the ritual that accompanies the recitation of a curing prayer (*reza*),[12] hence it is understandable why the wood should be considered adequate material for the manufacture of *figas*.[13]

Shakespeare uses the word 'fig' as a term of derision,[14] while phrases such as *fazer figa* or *dar figa* in Portugal have in the past been derogatory.[15] The *figa* gesture is considered obscene in a number of countries, particularly in Germany (where it may be employed to indicate a prostitute), Greece, Norway[16] and Persia. This strong link with Eros and the obscene no doubt stems from the *figa*'s clear representation of coition, and the reason for its use as a device to protect against forces of evil lies in its obscene nature.

The obscene and the grotesque are associated with the idea of protection from evil in a number of cultures. Certainly Exú, who protects and guards all entrances, and particularly the orifices of the body through which evil could penetrate, is represented by a mud phallus often standing in a bowl of *dendê* oil, or by a metal statue with an enormously accentuated phallus (this is particularly the case in Rio de Janeiro). The obscene and the grotesque are also traditional motifs in medieval Christian architecture, their main function being to protect the building and its occupants from the works of the devil.

Welsford, in a discussion of the possible origins of the institution of the court fool, refers to attempts to ascertain

> the date, origin and significance of certain small bronze and terra-cotta figures representing grotesques of various kinds: hunchbacks, pygmies, dwarfs, negroes, living skeletons, caricatures of ordinary men and women, who are usually represented as bald, or idiotic or with an exaggerated phallus.

She goes on to quote Professor Wace's article, 'Grotesques and the Evil Eye', in which he points out that:

> the workmanship of the bronzes is usually of the Imperial period . . . some may be intended not as portraits but as mascots.

Such images seem to have been popular all over the Graeco-Roman world, no doubt for the purpose referred to by Welsford, who states that:

> The possession of a hunchback, a bald head, or any striking deformity, is a good safeguard against this malignant influence [the evil eye] presumably because such misfortunes render one too wretched to excite either human or divine envy.[17]

However, fundamental to the notion of protecting from evil with representations of the obscene is the added dimension of the obscene gesture or object being a symbol of fertility. The fact that forces of evil, and particularly the force normally associated with the evil eye, can be repelled by such fertility symbols stems from the belief that infertility in all its forms (i.e. sterility in humans and animals, crop failures and so on) comes as a result of the power of the evil eye.[18] The best method of defence is a representation of a human sexual organ, or, better still, coition, that will serve to protect the subject's fertility from the damaging effects of the eye.

The term 'fertility' need not only be associated with offspring or crops in that all transformations that take place may be looked upon as being the result of the union of fundamental sources of energy, and it is the moment when transformation takes place that is considered the most dangerous. Little children and young animals are particularly prone to danger,[19] not so much because they are in a peculiarly defenceless state as because they are in the process of growing. In Brazil, a premature halt in the steady physical development of an infant is considered to be the work of the evil eye (C.2 and *passim*). Similarly, prolonged yawning fits, sleeplessness and continued crying in children are looked upon as being interruptions in the normal growing-up process caused by an evil eye. Other sources have quoted other instances when the evil eye may function at the moment when some form of transformation is taking place.[20]

A large majority of amulets made from animal teeth or horns are, at base, symbols of fertility, and as such are effective in repelling forces of evil. It is true that certain objects, such as a horn or a tooth, when used by themselves as amulets, impart the function they once possessed (defence) to the new owner, thereby protecting him from outside influences, but their further significance as fertility symbols must not be overlooked.[21] Horns and horn shapes have traditionally been associated with virility and the energy behind reproduction.[22] In Italy, it is common to wear sprigs of red coral (that resemble horns) as amulets to protect against the evil eye,[23] and Hausmann and Kriss-Rettenbeck (1966:200) give an illustration of one such amulet which has the majority of its individual branches ending in a carved *figa*.

The whole notion behind the crescent shape of the new moon (also a horn shape) is that it represents the beginning of a period of growth when the moon is endowed with all the power that links it to the movement of the tides, the female *menses*, the qualities of herbs and so forth. A curved tooth in isolation may protect because it is pointed and used to belong to a ferocious animal, but if it is joined with a similar tooth, it takes on the shape of the crescent moon and/or a pair of horns and becomes doubly powerful as a tool of protection (C.5).[24]

Cowrie shells (known in Brazil as *búzios*) are also endowed with a power to protect the wearer against the forces of the evil eye. They are not only common in Africa and Brazil as amulets, but also in Europe, where they are used as instruments of protection against forces of evil.[25] In Africa and in most Afro-Brazilian religions, cowrie shells are employed in an important system of divination and as such are looked upon as being endowed with special power.[26]

Their effectiveness as amulets may be linked to the strong resemblance which they bear to the vulva. Moreover, the shape of the shell and the slit in it can also be likened to a half-closed eye, which in itself would be sufficient to ward off any evil glances.[27] Certainly the eye and the vulva are similar, both in shape and in their common function as symbolic instruments of protection. Loewenthal, writing in 1972 (p. 832), says that 'until recently' female genitalia were portrayed in ornamental brass door knockers at the north entrance of Toledo cathedral, thus reinforcing the doorway which is the weakest point of defence. Amulets and talismans with the human eye incorporated in them have been and still are employed as means of protection.[28]

But if the vulva can protect it can also harm, as pointed out by Gifford (1958:142–3), who mentions a sixteenth-century Arabian manuscript that contains a warning that looking into the cavity of the vagina may be injurious to the eye. This dual nature of the female genitalia, whereby they can protect or harm, may be linked in some way with the widely held belief that a person with the power of overlooking also has the power to cure. The eye that harms is also the eye that can bring relief.[29]

Garlic is also ascribed qualities that link it to one or other of the two sexes, in that in Brazil a distinction is made between male garlic (*alho macho*) and female garlic (*alho fêmeo*), male garlic being long and thin and female garlic squat and rounded.[30] The sexual symbolism here is clear, but in the case of garlic it is only the *alho macho* which is used as a means of protection against the eye. A small clove is hidden behind the ear or included among the contents of a *patuá*.[31]

Other amulets in this category do not have sexual connotations, but are employed to ward off evil by other means. The pentangle[32] is very common in Brazil, both as an amulet which is worn on a chain or stamped on to such other amulets (thereby reinforcing them) as the base part of a *figa*.[33] It is also commonly found on the outside of the front door of dwelling houses,[34] and forms the basis for most cabbalistic signs drawn on the floor during certain curing rituals.[35]

Its widespread use as an instrument of protection is based on the fact that it embodies the efficiency of both the circle and the triangle, either in protecting the person who stands in the middle of it or imprisoning the devil within it so that he cannot escape to do harm to others. Risco (1961:80) quotes the legend in which Solomon was believed by the Arabs to have absolute power over both inferior and superior spirits who adored him and obeyed the sign. Those that revolted against him he imprisoned in pitchers sealed with his seal.[36] The pentangle's power resides in its five equal angles,[37] the pentagram contained at its centre and the fact that such a sign can be made in one movement without lifting the pencil from the paper. As soon as one of the angles is broken, the star not only loses its power to protect but becomes an instrument with which the sorcerer may do evil. Waite (1911:85, pl. V) gives a number of signs from the so-called *Fourth Book of Cornelius Agrippa* that represent the characters of evil spirits. The two examples reproduced here as Figures 1 and 2 are particularly significant in that they are versions of the regular pentangle that invite evil forces to enter.

FIGURE 1.

FIGURE 2.

The power of the regular pentangle resides particularly in each of the five angles. A common cure for snake-bite, for example, consists of drawing a pentangle on the ground and taking a handful of earth from each of its five points. The earth is then mixed with water and given to the patient to drink (C.2).[38] Sometimes it suffices to draw a pentangle over the affected area (C.2, C.5).[39] In Cachoeira, when transplanting a root of the *lança de Oxalá*, a pentangle should first be drawn on the earth and then the root planted in the middle. It is believed that a new shoot will ultimately appear at the tip of each of the five points (C.5).

The widespread use of the pentangle in Brazil stems particularly from the popularity it already enjoyed in Europe at the time of colonization and the fact that the Malé who went over to Brazil as slaves at the time of colonization had already been given it by the Arabs as an instrument of defence.[40] However, one of the reasons for its popularity among *Candomblé de caboclo* followers may be its similarity with the starfish, which has come to be adopted as an emblem for Yemanjá, the goddess of salt water (C.12, S.7).

Nickel steel rings[41] are also commonly worn, mainly to ward off disease, but if placed in the window inside a glass of water, the ring will protect the occupants of the house from the evil wind (see below, pages 106–8) (C.6, C.11, C.15). These rings appear to find their origin in Europe, and it is possible that their alleged powers of healing are linked to the fact that they are made of metal.[42] Metal is ascribed great powers in folk medicine, mainly because, as Eliade (1962:99) points out, there is a close connection between the art of the smith and the art of the shaman who heals. In the same way as the smith can transform ore into metals, so can the shaman transform illness into health.

Hildburgh (1940:246) mentions how rings that have been rubbed against the Caravaca cross protect the wearer from illness. Other writers mention the use of the ring in Europe as an amulet that protects against toothache (M'Clintock 1912:477), epilepsy (McKenzie 1927:200), paralysis, rheumatism, cramp, gout (Black 1883:172–7) and the plague (Thomas 1971:189). Rings worn in the ears cure weak or unhealthy eyes in Scotland (Maclagan 1902 1st edn 1972:134; Gifford 1958:87). A steel ring also serves to protect from evil forces. Vasconcellos (1882:101) records how steel rings are worn in Beira Alta to protect against witchcraft, those made on Maundy Thursday being particularly effective, while Hildburgh (1908:221) mentions the use of steel rings as amulets in Portugal to guard against the evil wind. Loewenthal (1972:33) gives an illustration of a Mediterranean belt buckle consisting of a hand with a ring on the little finger that served to protect the owner from evil.

In Brazil, nickel steel rings are commonly available in markets, with a wide variety of different cabbalistic signs imprinted on the broad face of the ring. The signs may vary from a pentangle to a series of dots, which are usually of an odd number and displayed in the same order as the different symbols representing the four suits on playing cards. Such rings may be worn as a general protection against all forms of illness, but they are considered particularly effective to combat an illness known popularly as *maniconia* (C.6, C.11). This is a type of rash that manifests itself in the form of black patches appearing on the skin, usually after the person concerned has been tense, nervous or angry. It is believed that if the patches appear over the heart, the patient is bound to die. Brazilian doctors I spoke to were unanimous in saying that *maniconia* was not an isolated illness, but that the term could have been chosen to refer to the patches that remain on the skin after certain varieties of syphilis.[43]

Herbs, nuts and seeds may also be employed in the manner of amulets to protect the wearer from evil. Three leaves of *guiné* or *arruda*[44] are sometimes worn behind the ear as a means of protection, and it is common to see *espada de Ogun*, *espada de Oxossi*, *pinhão roxo* or *vassourinha de Nossa Senhora* on the trays of street vendors. Sometimes the leaves are so arranged as to make a cross, and this is believed to render the leaves more powerful. Nutmeg and *umburana* worn on a string round the neck protects one against the evil wind, and the *fruta de São Cipriano*, collected in the proper ritual fashion, may be worn round the neck in the same manner. Other nuts/seeds which may be employed in the same way are *favico*, *bejerecum*, *fruta da ciência* (or *tontiça*).[45]

There is a more complex type of amulet that is known by two names:

(a) *patuá*, which is from the Tupi *patiguá* meaning hammock, basket or small box.[46] It has now come to mean a small leather or cloth bag.
(b) *breve*, which is from the Portuguese meaning brief. The term is now used to describe a small bag containing a brief prayer.[47]

Patuá and *breve* are now synonymous terms used to describe a small bag worn round the neck and supposedly containing a brief prayer or charm and other ingredients especially chosen to ward off the evil eye or to protect the wearer from an indisposition actually mentioned in the prayer.[48] They can be readily purchased in markets, but those made specifically for an individual are considered to be much more efficient.

Incorporated in the idea of the *patuá* is the same notion as underlies the North American Indian 'medicine bag'. The wearer remains fully in contact with those herbs and other substances that are generally believed to contain special powers to protect the body from all sources of danger. It is common to refer to such substances as being most efficacious to *fechar o corpo* (close/seal the body) in the sense of rendering it immune to hostile forces. In the same way as enormous powers were attributed to the 'medicine bag' by North American Indians,[49] so is the *patuá* looked upon as being an extremely powerful object that cannot fail to accomplish what its manufacturer stipulated when worn by its rightful owner. Ideally it retains its power throughout the lifetime of its owner (though at his death it will be useless to anybody else), but he must comply with taboos regarding its use. He should never touch it when he is *de corpo sujo*, nor must it ever be opened and the contents revealed. If these taboos are not carefully followed, the *patuá* loses all its power.[50]

The use of amulets consisting of small leather bags filled with leaves and similar objects has continued to be a common practice among the Yoruba.[51] Sometimes the container consists of a horn filled with the different substances, thus contributing the additional power of the horn shape to the amulet.[52] In Brazil, the contents of *patuás* vary considerably in accordance with the preferences and beliefs of the maker, and since most prescriptions obtained included *pemba preparada*, it follows that the maker of the *patuá* should include in leaf form one or more of the herbs he uses in the manufacture of *pemba*. Querino (1938:97–8) maintains that the *patuá* should contain something belonging to the wearer's *orixá*, but I did not find this to be the case.[53]

Prescriptions obtained for *patuás* are as follows:

A *abre caminhos*
alho macho
dandá
guiné
vencetudo
pemba
[I.2]

B *pemba* by itself
[C.4]

C *bejerecum*
dandá (preferably picked on Good Friday)
(jet) *figa*
(*arruda*) *figa*
pemba (sometimes)
[C.5]

D One leaf of *abre caminhos* is placed in a red bag on one side of which must be attached a cross made of *alecrim*, on the other a pentangle sewn with red cotton. The cord on which the *patuá* is suspended should also be red. The colour red is significant because it is the colour of Yansan, the goddess of the thunderbolt, who can withstand all danger, including the spirits of the dead (*egun*). If the usual taboos are not followed, Yansan may send punishment whether or not she is the *orixá* who controls the person wearing the *patuá*. [C.11]

One prescription was obtained for a *patuá* specifically designed to ward off any illness:

E Any leaf that comes under the control of Omolú, especially *catinga de porco* and *jurema preta*. Include with a piece of rock salt and a clove of male garlic in a square of black material. The material should then be gathered by the corners and tied with one long piece of straw. [C.6]

The above contents are usually, though not necessarily always, wrapped in a prayer or charm. Those that I came across were, without exception, handwritten, though Maynard Araújo (1961:68) maintains that the prayer is more commonly printed than handwritten.

The practice of wearing a prayer or charm, or any sacred text around the neck, was common both in medieval Europe and among the Moslem tribes (particularly the Malé and Hausa) who were sent to Brazil as slaves. Black (1883:165–71) quotes various examples of charms carried on one's person to ward off the evil eye and various illnesses, while Lis Quibén (1949:489–90, quoting López) describes a small bag containing the four gospels in Latin, worn by children either round the neck or hidden in clothing, as a means of protection against the evil eye.[54] The *Enchiridion of Pope Leo III* (a textbook on occult practices styled on the grimoires) contains instructions to its owner that it should be kept in a bag of new leather and carried as far as practicable on his person.[55]

The Malé were particularly well known in Brazil for their custom of wearing quotations from the Koran written on paper, small pieces of wood or other suitable substances, and hidden inside a small leather bag. These bags were called *mandingas*, and the Malé themselves came to be known as *mandingueiros*.[56] Such amulets are still common in West Africa, where they are traded particularly by the Hausa.[57] However, it is most unlikely that any of the *patuás* at present in use in Brazil should contain prayers in Arabic, because the Malé and Hausa groups have been broken up, the majority having become associated with *Candomblé de caboclo*.[58] The efficacy of a *patuá*, moreover, dies with its owner, so the traditional-styled ones should by now have disappeared.[59]

Prayers for inclusion in *patuás* are rarely originally made up by the maker. Many of them are, in fact, very similar to those readily available in such publications as the *Livro Antigo e Verdadeiro de São Cipriano*. C.4 becomes possessed by her *orixá*, and then she chooses the appropriate prayer out of any of the cheap publications containing such prayers, the Bible, or a priest's breviary. The prayer is then copied out and included in the pertinent *patuá*. Usually, in this case, the type of prayer chosen will be in accord with the patient's own *orixá*, so a patient with a female *orixá* will be given a prayer that entreats the intercession of a female saint. The opposite occurs if the patient belongs to a male *orixá*.

Prayers are usually directed towards a Catholic saint, though occasionally the African equivalent will be invoked. One informant, C.2, mentioned that he knew specific prayers that governed all usual illnesses, and the appropriate one would be selected to suit the occasion. He would not part with the prayers, though I suspect they may be identical to those curing prayers that cover a whole range of illnesses that will be discussed in the next chapter.

Cascudo (1962:I, 135), however, mentions how some *patuás* were, when opened, found to contain banalities and obscenities, but he gives no examples. Campos (1967:115–16) gives the following charms to assist parturition:

Me and my horse doing well; whoever wants to give birth let her do so for this reason, and, if she can't let her die of congestion.

Let me have shelter, and my horse. Let the ass give birth, don't let it bother me.[60]

I came across nothing similar to these among prayers that may be included in *patuás*. A random inspection of marketed *patuás*, however, revealed that the majority contained either blank pieces of paper or small cuttings from printed prayers in the Catholic style, cut out in such a haphazard manner as to render them meaningless. None of them contained any complete prayer. It is significant, on the other hand, that these marketed *patuás* are not normally purchased and worn by people who seriously wish to protect themselves from the forces of evil. Marketed *patuás* appeal mainly to tourists, and are never taken very seriously by initiates or serious cult followers.

The following prayers are not, to my knowledge, included in the cheap publications usually owned by *curandeiros*. It is intended merely to transcribe and comment very briefly on prayers normally included in *patuás*, since a fuller discussion of the principal characteristics of prayers will be given in the next chapter.

The first appears to be an orthodox prayer in the Catholic tradition, though I was assured that the 'guardian angel' referred not to the Catholic guardian angel but to the *orixá*. The same is true in the final sentence of the second prayer, in which 'guide' must be looked upon as being a synonym of *orixá*.

1 I surrender myself to Jesus, to His most holy cross, to the most holy sacrament, and to the three relics which are contained therein. Most Holy Mary, be ever by my side. Guardian angel, guard me, deliver me from Satan's cunning ways and practices. [I.2]

2 Christ and S. Jorge in times of trouble wearied by their enemies. May the wearer of this prayer have the strength to soften tyrannical hearts, Lord Jesus, by my faith in S. Claúdio, Aleluia. I trample the hearts of my enemies beneath my feet. S. Jorge is my guide. [I.2]

The Catholic saint most commonly invoked for assistance is Saint George, but he is very clearly linked all the time with Oxossi (*orixá* of the hunt), as revealed in the following prayer, which contains both Catholic and African names:

3 Lord, may my body always remain sealed and immune to any ill brought about by man. I ask that my enemies be always confounded when they try to harm me. I ask that my body be always protected from any arm or firearm. May the lance of S. Jorge to whom I am devoted be always at the ready to defend me, and may the blood never flow from my body, and may my enemies find themselves impotent when they try to destroy me, may Oxossi's sword be ever above my head to avoid any evil-doing. [I.6]

The terms of address used are deliberately vague (e.g. *fulano*[61] in No. 4, which follows) so that the *patuá* may have the same powers against any evil wisher:

4 *Fulano*, sorcerer Cobé, sorcerer without enlightenment or faith, before you were born the child Jesus was born. My weakness before you and your strength I hold down beneath my left foot. *Fulano*, you are powerless against me, and always will be, for I have the three persons of the Most Holy Trinity on my side. In the name of Jesus. Ave Maria. [C.6]

The statement 'before you were born the child Jesus was born' is repeated again and again whenever an evil spirit becomes incorporated in a medium during a spirit session, and ultimately serves to drive it away. The notion that forces of evil can be overcome if trampled under the left foot is common and will be seen again in the ritual *trabalho* (see below, page 116).

Another way of overcoming evil forces is to establish one's superiority by means of stating antitheses:

5 *Fulano*, you are bronze, I am steel; you are fire, I am water.[62] If you bear any evil, any perverse wishes against me, I, *Fulano*, with the powers of God, of heaven, of the earth and sea, will break you down, dissolve you before my very eyes. You must be humbled and your powers shattered by me, by the power of God and the Virgin Mary. Amen. [I.2]

6 Covered by the mantle of Our Lady the Guide, I shall walk and not walk, and meet my enemies. They will do me no harm nor will I harm them. I shall walk and not walk. I shall find a shrine. It was the angel Gabriel who met Our Lady and greeted her praying Ave Maria. The hand of the Almighty shall fall on whoever wishes to do me evil. May he be struck as still as stone while I, poor sinner, try to walk in God's ways, Amen.[63] [I.2]

A person's inviolability may also be stressed by employing a form based on ritual chanting, as in the final lines of the next prayer.

7 Forward Jesus, peace and guide, I commend myself to God and the Virgin Mary my mother and to the twelve Apostles my brothers. I shall walk by day and night, my body surrounded and defended by the arms of S. Jorge. My body will not be captured or wounded, nor will my blood

be spilt. I shall be as free as Jesus Christ was nine months in the Virgin's womb. My enemies will have eyes, but not see me. They will have mouths and be speechless. They will have feet, but not catch up with me. They will have hands but do me no harm. (Whoever wears this prayer round his neck will not be harmed by his enemies.) [C.2]

Formulas of this type are common in such prayers and are to be found all over Brazil. Birnfeld (1951:60), for example, gives:

Free me Jesus, from my enemies, if they have eyes, may they not see me, if they have ears, may they not hear me, if they have hands, may they not hit me, if they have mouths, may they not speak to me, if they have arms, may they not wound me; may the mouths of dogs and wolves be sealed to me, likewise the mouths of my enemies. May I remain in peace and concord. Amen.[64]

Before the *patuá* is sealed, the maker should make repeated signs of the cross over it with his right hand while requesting out loud all the *orixás* to join together and give strength to the *orixá* or saint who controls the prayer inside the *patuá*. This request takes the form of a spontaneous prayer, an example of which is transcribed here:

8 My glorious Father, I implore, and call on God and ask you to give strength to all the *orixás*, enlightenment to him to whom this prayer is made, he being S. Jorge, that he may be a guide and protector to all those who use this, may he seal their bodies, lead them out of temptation, shattering the forces of their enemies, that they may never have strength to bring about any evil-doing against those who use this. With the power of God and the Virgin Mary. Praised be Our Lord Jesus Christ. May he give strength and health to those who use this; be it as a protection; be it to seal the body, and be it for them to acquire anything in life they may require for their spiritual development. [I.2]

In the majority of cases, the *patuá* is now ready for use, but C.4 mentioned that, before allowing it to be used, it should be taken to church by the maker and lifted up in the right hand in the direction of the altar at the moment when the priest elevates the host.

CHAPTER X

THE REZA (CURING PRAYER)

Certain prayers, usually those that cover fairly minor complaints (e.g. *verrugas* = warts) are usually recited by ordinary individuals (often the patient himself), but in more serious cases it is considered that a cure will be more likely if someone who specializes in such things is consulted. C.13 earned his livelihood entirely by reciting prayers for ill people, and was known locally as a *rezador* or *benzedor* (man who prays/blesses). However, it is considered that the cure will be considerably more effective and speedy if the prayer is recited by a *pai* or *mãe de santo*, especially in cases involving the evil eye and/or the ill wind. The *pai* or *mãe de santo* in such cases recites the prayer in the normal fashion and never falls into the trance state at any stage during the ritual.

Most prayers are accompanied by certain ritual acts, the main one being the gentle brushing of certain leaves in the shape of a cross against the patient's body, or that particular part of the body where the illness is located. This is very akin to the idea behind *sacudida*, but in a *reza* the leaves do no more than just touch the skin as opposed to being brought down heavily on the body. Moreover, for a *reza* it is only necessary for the *curandeiro* to hold three leaves of any one plant in his hand, while for a *sacudida* he is required to hold definite numbers of whole sprigs that may withstand prolonged heavy treatment. Any other prescribed ritual will be pointed out at the time of transcribing the prayer.

All informants stressed that any herb may be used during a *reza* (though I.2 did not include herbs that belong to Exú). There are, however, certain herbs that informants single out from others as being particularly efficacious for use during a *reza*. Analysis of them shows that the majority are fairly evenly distributed among all the *orixás* (see Table 9). It should be borne in mind, however, that two of the herbs, *arruda* and *manjericão*, have traditionally been used for *rezas* in Portugal and Spain, and this may be the principal factor behind their continued use in Brazil rather than their attachment to any particular *orixá*.

Whereas informants are quick to point out the various herbs that may be used during a *reza*, the fact is that only five are used all the time. These are: *arruda*, *guiné*, *manjericão*, *pinhão roxo*, *vassourinha de Nossa Senhora*. It may be significant that all these herbs come under the control, either

Table 9. Number of herbs used during a *reza* under each *orixá*.

Orixá	*Number of Herbs Controlled*
Yemanjá	10
Omolú	8
Oxun	7
Naná	7
Yansan	6
Ogun	6
Oxossi	4
Exú	3
Oxalá	3
Xangô	2

wholly or partially, of Omolú, the one exception being *manjericão*. However, *manjericão* is controlled in part by Naná, a feminine equivalent of Omolú, who is extremely close to him in every way. She is considered to be very old, and in one of the myths is depicted as the mother of Omolú. It is stressed, however, that the practice of using *manjericão* and *arruda* may not be based on their association with any particular *orixá* but on their traditional employment in Europe to accompany a *reza*.

It is common to have one or more of the five herbs listed here growing either in the confines of the *caboclo* cult houses or in front of a whole row of dwelling houses for the use of all the occupants. Ordinary *caboclo* cult followers who are not members of the priestly hierarchy tend to take their own herbs of their own choice to the *pai* or *mãe de santo* when requiring a *reza*, and they inevitably choose one of the standard five herbs usually found growing near their houses since it is very rare for people outside the priestly hierarchy to have a particularly deep knowledge of plant lore.

As in the case of *sacudida*, the patient stands opposite an open door all the way through the ritual. Some *pais* or *mães de santo* actually prefer to conduct the *reza* inside the *pejí* (I.3, I.4, I.6, C.2, C.3, C.9, S.2). The prayer is recited in a low voice at very high speed so that only one or two words may be caught. Fast recitation was common in all cases observed, and informant C.3 mentioned that the reason for this was to ensure that the prayer was recited without the *curandeiro* being distracted in any way that might make him falter or make a mistake. Were he to do so, he would have to start again from the beginning.[1] S.5 observed that a mistake in the recitation of prayers for the evil eye implies that the evil inside the patient is beginning to affect the *curandeiro*. For this reason, it is common for the person reciting the prayer to keep a small piece of *dandá* or *alho macho* in the left side of his or her mouth. C.2 only ever conducts a *reza* while wearing his *patuá*, and C.6 makes a cross with a clove of *alho macho* over the pulse in each wrist before commencing the *reza*. All informants maintained that it was common to feel the force of evil when reciting a *reza* to cure the evil wind and/or the evil eye, and that it was for this reason that some protective measure should be taken.

It has been pointed out elsewhere how most cultures recall myths, and how these myths may have enormous significance for the whole community:

> myth is thought to express the *absolute truth*, because it narrates a *sacred history* . . . Being *real* and *sacred*, the myth becomes exemplary, and consequently *repeatable*, for it serves as a model, and by the same token as a justification, for all human actions. In other words, a myth is a *true history* of what came to pass at the beginning of Time, and one which provides the pattern for human behaviour.[2] [Eliade 1972:23]

Many myths refer back to a moment in time when man's condition was paradisiacal, and many creation myths go on to describe how some form of catastrophe occurred shortly after creation which resulted in man's forfeiting his paradisiacal existence for the one he leads at present. It is common among many cultures to attempt to re-create the state of paradise such as existed at the beginning of the world, and this is done primarily by the repetition of myth. By imitating the actions of the god who created the world, it is believed that the person in question can leave his current dimension and re-enter the dimension of perfection that existed before the catastrophe occurred. Then, as he emerges out of paradise into his familiar world, he is a new man and feels refreshed. Many informants in Brazil mentioned how, on emerging from the trance state in which they had been possessed by their *orixás*, they felt rested and refreshed. This feeling was once described with the verb *limpar* (to clean), *O orixá limpa o medium* ('The *orixá* cleanses the medium') (C.2).

One method of treating illness among many cultures is to recite myth and to re-enact the actions of the gods. It is believed that, by so doing, the patient will transcend the present moment, be transported to the beginning of time and finally return to the present in full health. By being transported back to the moment of creation, he is able to be created again. The notion of death and rebirth that is common to most acts of transformation may be seen, therefore, in the treatment of illness. Reichel-Dolmatoff (1971:177–8) describes the treatment of illness as follows:

In principle, an illness is imagined as a wrapping, a thin black cape that envelops the patient and must be broken in some manner to accomplish the cure. Obviously, this cape represents the placenta, and the sick person himself is compared with a foetus. An effective cure consists then in producing a birth. What is sought is to rupture the envelope and to reincorporate the patient into normal life. There is one single word—*mahsári*—meaning to cure and to be born.

One of the main characteristics of most of the curing prayers currently in use in Brazil is that they belong to the tradition of myth. They often tell a story which is about the patron saint or saints of the illness that is to be cured, though mention of any saint, even a fictitious one, appears to be quite acceptable. Sometimes the prayer takes the form of a conversation conducted between the saints and Jesus Christ[3] in which Christ asks the saints where they are going. When they reply that they are on their way to cure a certain illness, Jesus Christ tells them the ingredients with which to cure. The prayer then often ends with a recitation by both patient and *curandeiro* of one or more of the standard Catholic prayers (e.g. *Pater Noster*, *Ave Maria*, *Salve Regina*).

Some informants make distinctions between which standard prayers should be said depending on the sex of the patient. If the patient is a man, the *Ave Maria* or *Salve Regina* should be recited, if a woman, the *Pater Noster* or *Gloria Patri* (I.1, C.6, C.11, C.14, S.1).

The meeting and/or conversation as reported in the prayer is usually historically fictitious, but both patient and *curandeiro* must believe that what is being recited is the truth, for without such faith it is thought that no cure is possible. *São as palavras de Deus, e Deus cura tudo* ('They are the words of God and God cures everything') (C.6).

The examples of prayers transcribed below are English translations of the original Portuguese:

Azia, mal de azia (heartburn)

1 Santa Iria has three daughters. One spins, another sews and the other cures *mal d'azia*.[4] [S.1]

Campainha caída

This is an inflammation of the throat believed to be caused by a change in position of the Adam's apple, known as *campainha*—hence *campainha caída*, fallen Adam's apple.

2 As the priest robes and unrobes and goes up to the altar so *campainha caída* must you return to your place. [C.7]

3 Open doors facing the sea, *campainha caída* return to your place with the keys of the sanctuary accompanying you.[5] [C.13]

While the prayer is being recited, the patient must insert his finger in his mouth and press upwards on the palate while the person reciting pulls the patient's hair with one hand while brushing the leaves in the form of a cross over his Adam's apple (C.13). C.7, however, omits pulling the hair.[6]

Cobreiro or *empinge* (shingles)

It is commonly believed that this illness is caused by an insect or animal such as a toad or lizard either crawling over a piece of clothing which is subsequently worn, or actually coming into physical contact with the skin. The rash is looked upon as covering the area contaminated by the animal. It is believed that, if the two ends meet, the patient will die (I.2 and *passim*).[7] Different rituals accompany the curing prayers: a solution of water and salt is prepared in a saucer. The leaf is then dipped in the saucer and crosses are described over the affected area.

4 I came from Rome on a pilgrimage saying prayers for *cobreiro de cobraria*, *cobreiro* from toads, *cobreiro* from spiders, *cobreiro* from snakes, *cobreiro* from lizards, *cobreiro* from all harmful creatures, with a green twig and cold water, with God's power and that of the Virgin. [C.13]

The following prayer is accompanied by the same gestures, except that the leaf used must be *vassourinha de Nossa Senhora* and the mixture made with three pinches of salt.

5 I came from Rome on a pilgrimage saying prayers for *cobreiro* from snakes, lizards, toads, and spiders, with a green twig and cold water, with God's power and that of the Virgin. [S.1]

In another case, the liquid is pure vinegar, and after use the leaf must be left in the sun to dry. The letters JMJ, standing for Jesus, Maria, José (Jesus, Mary, Joseph), may then be written in ink over the affected area.[8]

6 My Santo Antonio, as this leaf is virgin so is this illness; as this leaf dies so may this illness. [S.5]

I.2 gave the following prayer, which should be recited three times every day for three days:

7 I come from Rome on a pilgrimage curing *cobreiro* caused by animals and insects, with green twigs and cold water, with God's power and that of the Virgin. [I.2]

The prayer may also be accompanied by a symbolic cutting, the *cobreiro* itself being metaphorically seen as an animal with a head and a tail. Crosses are made over the affected area with the stalk of a *mamona* leaf while saying:

8 Bold *cobreiro*, I cut off your head. [C.6]

A small piece is then cut off the stalk at the end where the leaf used to grow. Then the stalk is again brushed over the area while saying:

Bold *cobreiro*, I cut off your tail.

A small piece is then cut off the other end of the stalk. The above is repeated three times, followed by:

The following words I dedicate to São Martim and São Gonçalo.

There next follows the *Pater Noster* in Portuguese. All the pieces are then threaded on to a string which is tied to form a loop and hung on a tree (C.6).

Another example of symbolic cutting involves the reciter holding a bunch of *coerana* leaves at one end while the patient holds the other. The reciter cuts the leaves during the following dialogue:

9 PATIENT: What are you doing?
RECITER: I am cutting off head, body and tail. [I.2]

This is repeated three times, then the following is said while the affected area is brushed with *vassourinha de Nossa Senhora* steeped in vinegar:

I came from Rome on a pilgrimage saying prayers for *cobreiro de cobraria*, be it from a toad, a snake, lizards big or small, a spider, with God's power and that of Senhor São Bento I cast you out of here, with God's power and that of the Virgin.

The conversation technique is common in many *cobreiro* prayers.[9] Sometimes the conversation is between two saints,[10] though more often it is between a saint and Jesus Christ.[11]

Dor de cabeça (headache)

I.2 uses prayers for the evil eye to cure headaches, and C.13 uses the same prayer as for *Sol na cabeça* (see below, page 104ff.).

The following, however, is used exclusively for headaches, despite the fact that the sun is mentioned as a possible cause.

10 Flaviano and Lauriano went to a spring called the mount to pluck a leaf of mountain olive, to say prayers for headache, for *chaqueta*,[12] for *maleta*,[13] from the sun, from the night air. Come back Lauriano and Flaviano, join temple with temple. When Noah's ark falls and rises the patient's headache will go with the water of the mountain spring, Jesus, Mary and Joseph. So be it. Amen.[14] [S.1]

Dor de dentes (toothache)

Guiné leaves (preferably) should be brushed over the area affected to the accompaniment of this prayer:

11 São Manso, tamer, who tamed the bulls and the fierce lions, so must I tame this toothache which is bedevilling me. The blood flows, the

heart beats, the pain of this tooth disappears in the waves of the sacred sea. [C.6]

The majority of curing prayers for toothache, however, usually refer to Saints Pelonha[15] or Pedro, who are often depicted sitting on a stone, as in the following example:

12 Santa Pelonha was seated on a cold stone. The Virgin came along asking: What are you doing Pelonha, sitting on that cold stone? It's toothache and neuralgia, my Lady. Pelonha, as I carry on my arm this child that was born of me, in God's name I swear your toothache will pass away. By the rising sun and the setting moon, by our Lord Jesus Christ may Pelonha's toothache leave her.[16] [C.13]

The reference to the sun or the moon is common, reflecting the notion that toothache may be related to the movements of celestial bodies.[17]

Engasgo (choking fits)

Prayers for *engasgo* are usually very short on account of the immediate danger which faces the patient. The reciter makes crosses with his thumb over the patient's throat.

13 Good man, bad woman, old rush mat, bone in the throat. [C.11]

The prayer refers back to a legend in which Jesus Christ (S.4 stipulates Jesus Christ and Saint Peter) arrived disguised as a beggar at a house and asked for food and lodging. He was well received by the husband, but the wife grumbled, refused to give him any of the chicken she was preparing for the family dinner, and sent him outside to the yard to sleep on an old mat. The following morning, after she had sent the visitor away, she choked herself on one of the chicken bones. Her husband went in search of the beggar, who taught him the prayer and revealed his true identity (C.5).[18]

Prayers directed exclusively to São Braz order him to clear the patient's throat by making the obstacle go up or down where appropriate:

14 Bishop São Braz, Slave of Christ, go up or down, obey.[19] [I.1]

C.13 gave the following prayer, which does not fit into either of the categories already given:

15 I saw our Lord of Nazareth you, the joy of those who have faith. This throat will heal, this choking will end. With these prayers your throat will be cleansed. God bless you with this cross and forgive our sins, oh Jesus. [C.13]

Erisipela (erysipelas)

Prayers for *erisipela* are usually accompanied by the application of olive oil with herbs (I.1), a feather (I.2, C.5),[20] or esparto grass (C.1).[21] Ott (1957:II, 42) points out how certain prayers have been adapted to suit local conditions, hence, in Bahia, where sheep are rare, sheep's wool is not used. The words of the prayer, however, which often contain the ingredients for the cure, tend not to change. I.2, who supplied Prayer 16, underlined the importance of reciting it *verbatim*, but stipulated the use of a feather to apply the oil, and not sheep's wool as mentioned in the prayer.[22]

Sometimes the patient is required during recitation of the prayer to sit with the foot corresponding to the side of his body in which the disease has the greater hold resting on the back of a tortoise. He should press firmly on the tortoise so as not to allow it to move (I.2).[23]

Prayers for *erisipela* may take the form of a conversation between Saints Peter and Paul and Jesus Christ on the road to Rome. It is very common to give synonyms for *erisipela* and other illnesses through a fear that mentioning the name of the illness may be dangerous and entice it to stay longer in the body. Synonyms for *erisipela* will be in italics in the text.

16 Pedro Paulo went to Rome. Pedro Paulo came from Rome. Jesus Christ met them. Jesus Christ asked them: —Pedro Paulo, what is going on in Rome? —Much *zipole* and many are dying of it. —Pedro Paulo, return, go and cure the sick. —With what, Lord? —With olive oil, live sheep's wool, with the grace of God and the Virgin Mary will you cure. [I.2]

17 Pedro Paulo went to Rome and met Jesus. —Where are you going, Pedro and Paulo? —I'm going to cure *mal de monte*, Lord —With what

do you cure? —With oil, Lord, and the three words of the Most Holy Trinity and the twelve apostles who accompanied you. [C.6]

18 Pedro and Paulo went to Rome. On the way they met Jesus Christ. He asked —What's going on there, Pedro Paulo? They replied —*mal de monte*, Lord. —Go back. Pedro Paulo. Go and say prayers for that illness so it never returns. —With what shall I pray, Lord? —Olive oil. Oil will cure you with the power of God and the Virgin Mary.[24] [S.1]

One other prayer records a conversation between the reciter and three Marys:

19 I was sitting on a beach and three Marias came along, Maria Marta, Maria Madalena and Maria Mother of Jesus, asking: —What are you doing on this beach? —Saying prayers for *mal do monte* and *mal da praia*. — Pray in the name of the Father, of the Son and of the Holy Spirit. [C.13]

Another type of prayer traces the progess of the illness as it is forced out of the body towards the sea:

20 *Isipra*, *isipela*, *isipelão*, *zipra*, *zipelão*, go from the marrow to the bone, from bone to flesh, from flesh to skin, from skin to the ebbing tide.[25] [I.3]

The following version, however, gives a list of synonyms for the illness, all of which are then thrown in the sea:

21 I saw our Lord of Nazareth, You, the joy of those who have faith, *Mal de monte*, *mal da praia* and the wretched *esipelas*, and the wretched *esipelas* which I throw in the waves. [C.13]

Espinhela caída

There is no direct equivalent of *espinhela caída* in scientific medical terminology, and the name may be applied to any pain in the chest, back or stomach that stops a person holding himself fully upright. The term *espinhela caída* may be applied to a whole range of different indispositions for which scientific medicine has separate names, but it refers most commonly to a pain localized round the base of the rib-cage.[26] *Espinhela caída* is regarded as being very serious since it may lead to other illnesses such as tuberculosis, cancer, liver and heart complaints (C.13), or to prolonged restricted breathing (C.6). I.2 uses one and the same prayer (No. 22) for *espinhela caída*, backache and any form of serious indisposition such as coronary thrombosis or tuberculosis. All informants agreed that *espinhela caída* may be inflicted by the evil eye or come on the ill wind.

Diagnosis consists of measuring certain parts of the body and comparing the measurements with other parts. It is believed that the person concerned has contracted *espinhela caída* if there is any disparity between the two measurements. The most usual technique is to measure with a piece of string from the elbow to the tip of the little finger, and then to stretch the resulting length of string from one shoulder to another. If the string is too long, the person concerned is believed to be suffering from *espinhela caída* (I.2, C.6, C.11).[27]

This procedure most probably finds its origins in the ancient practice of girdle-measuring in Europe. Thomas (1971:184) quotes a document of 1566 which describes a similar method:

she measureth the girdle or band of any such persons being sick or haunted, from her elbow to her thumb, craving God for Saint Charity's sake that if [they] be haunted with a fairy, yea or no, she may know, and saith that if it be so the band will be shorter and her cubit will reach further than commonly it doth.

And he goes on to conclude:

The assumption behind it was that the presence of an evil spirit ('fairy') would reflect itself in the inconstancy of the measured length.

A similar procedure is mentioned by Gifford (1958:87–8) with reference to the Southern Slavs:

The victim stands with arms outstretched at shoulder level while the good witch, muttering magic words, measures with twine the distance from left heel to chin, from right middle fingertip to left middle fingertip, from left heel to right hand, and from right heel to left hand. Differences in measurement give diagnosis and prognosis, and cutting the twine with a knife after each measurement cuts away the sickness.

In Brazil, it is believed that an essential part of tissue has become dislodged and 'fallen' from its rightful place, and the prayers often refer to 'raising' it to its former position.

22 When God walked the world he raised *espinhela caída*. Open chest, open rib-cage, he raised with the help of God and the Virgin Mary. Amen.[28] [I.2]

Sometimes the reciter of the prayer stands behind the patient and pushes together both sides of the rib-cage (C.6, C.11, C.13, I.8). The expressions 'open chest' and 'open rib-cage' refer to a possible collapse in the structure of the rib-cage:

23 Pedro and Paulo came from Rome. On the way they met Jesus Christ. Jesus Christ asked: —Where have you come from Pedro and Paulo? —Lord, from Rome. —And what did you find there? —Lord I found open chests, I found open rib-cages, twisted ribs and twisted breastbones. [C.13]

Other prayers refer to the windows of a house facing the sea, but it is not clear whether this is intended to make the *espinhela caída* sympathetically turn towards and ultimately disappear in the sea, or whether the house should be an example to the *espinhela caída* of something solid and unshakeable.

24 São Pedro made his house with four windows, two facing the sea and two facing the land. So *espinhela*, I wish to raise you by S. Pedro and S. Paulo and all the saints in the heavenly courts. So *espinhela* return to your place. [I.2]

25 I met S. Pedro and S. Paulo on the road. Jesus asks: —Where are you going Pedro and Paulo? —To cure *espinhela caída*. —How do you cure, Pedro and Paulo? —I have my house with four windows towards the sea. So *espinhela caída* go back to your place.[29] [C.6]

Another example of sympathy may be found in the type of prayer that requests the *espinhela* to return to its original position as effortlessly as the priest ascends the altar:

26 As the priest robes and rerobes and ascends the altar, so *espinhela caída* go back to your place.[30] [I.1]

Frouxo (haemorrhage, flux)

Frouxo is a wide term that is applied to bleeding of all forms, particularly abnormal menstruation, nose bleeds and cuts.[31]

Prayers simply call upon the blood to coagulate:

27 Blood, be contained as it was contained in our Lord Jesus Christ.[32] Blood, stay in the veins as our Lord Jesus Christ had at the Supper. Blood, stay in the body as our Lord Jesus Christ stayed in the Garden.[33] [S.1]

Ingua (bubo)

Ingua can be cured by pointing a knife at a large star in the night sky and saying:

28 O star, this *íngua* said, may you die and it live. I say may it die and you live.[34] [I.2]

A cross over the affected areas should be made with the knife during the second half of the prayer. Paula (1952:19), who gives a similar prayer, says that the cure should be effected preferably during the wane of the moon and directed at a star that is shortly to set over the horizon, thus taking the illness with it.

Another method consists of pointing a knife or a finger at a stick in the wall of the house (the houses of the poor are usually built of wattle and daub) and saying either:

29 One, two, three, out with the *íngua*. [C.7]

or

30 Three, two, one, no more *íngua*.[35] [S.1]

Other sources say that the patient should touch the hearthstone, stay near the fire (Barroso 1949:441; Maynard Araújo 1958:141; Lis Quibén 1945:295) or point to the tiles on the roof (Gouveia 1926:24).

Mau olhado, olho mal; quebranto (*e*) (evil eye; overlooking)

The evil eye falls into two distinct categories. First, there is what is known as *quebranto* or *quebrante*, known in English as 'overlooking', which is a force which disrupts of its own accord and which is never deliberately conjured up by anybody. Usually it emanates from some person who happens from birth to possess the power to bring misfortune on others without deliberately wishing to. The word *quebranto*, meaning literally a breaking, implies no sense of evil whatsoever. Similarly, the Greek name, *baskania* (βασκανία) implies no notion of evil in that it means simply envy, and the Portuguese *invidia*, also meaning envy, is often used as a synonym for *quebranto*. It is commonly believed that words of praise may be a veiled form of envy, hence many indispositions are attributed to the fact that the patient may have been the subject of some recent adulation. This is particularly relevant in the case of small children, who are extremely prone to *quebranto* (see above, page 76).

The second category is known in Portuguese as *mau olhado*, *olhado* or *olho mau*(*l*) (evil eye), and this refers to the deliberate infliction of some evil force by one person on another. It is seen as a force of evil that is put on a person with the deliberate intention of disrupting the normal functioning of his body.

Prayers for the evil eye tend to make no clear-cut distinction between *quebranto* and *olho mau*, it being quite common to mention the two distinct varieties in the same prayer. Illnesses brought by overlooking and the evil eye are legion, and may range from a minor indisposition, such as a headache, to stunted growth in infants and serious illnesses that result in death. Because of this, prayers to counteract the influence of the evil eye may be recited before the prayers for the illness in question (C.13, S.5, S.6, S.7). C.13, who was consulted for a cure for chronic erysipelas, diagnosed first the evil eye and recited the appropriate prayer, followed by the prayer for erysipelas.[36] *Pais* and *mães de santo*, however, usually consult their *orixá* in such cases, and if the verdict turns out to be that the patient's illness stems directly from the evil eye, then only prayers to cure the evil eye are recited. It is considered in these cases that the illness will disappear as soon as the evil force has been expelled (I.2, I.3, I.6, I.7, C.2, C.5, C.6).

A common method of diagnosing the evil eye is to drop three drops of olive oil into a saucer of water. If they cannot be seen floating on the surface of the water, the person is believed to be a victim of the evil eye.

The herbs most commonly employed are *vassourinha de Nossa Senhora*, *arruda* and *guiné* (I.2 and *passim*), though S.1 and C.11 prefer *Maria preta* and *São Gonçalinho*.[37]

One type of prayer establishes the reciter's superiority over the evil force inside the patient. The evil force is compared to iron, while the reciter is compared to steel:

31 Take away what you brought. God bless me with His most holy cross. God defend me from *maus olhos* and *maus olhados*, from all the evil wished on me. You are iron, I am steel, you are the devil and I confound you in the name of the Father, Son and Holy Ghost.[38] [I.2]

Other prayers list the various means by which the patient might have become afflicted by the evil eye.

32 God made you and raised you. God was born in the Virgin's womb. *Fulano*, they used two to put it on you, I'll pray over you with three,[39] and the Father, Son and Holy Ghost. *Olhados* which were cast over you, whether when you were eating, when you were drinking, when you were lying down, or when you were getting up, *olhado de mofina*,[40] *olhado de quebrante*, whether when you were at work, when you were labouring, when you were at your daily bread, whether cast by a thin man, or a fat man, whether you were walking, whether you were hard at work, by day, or evening, with the power of God and the Virgin Mary, let them (the *olhados*) be cast out into the waters of the sea. [C.13]

33 Maria, why did you let the *olhado* be put on you? Be it by an ugly woman, or a thin one, or a fat one, or a pretty one, be it in your walking, or in your look, be it good, or bad, whether it makes you happy, or sad, be it in your conversation, or your eating, or drinking, get out of here *olhos mal*, away to the waves of the holy sea, where no cock crows nor hen, to where you cannot see the sun set, with the power of God and our Lady Mother the Virgin. Get out of here *quebrante* with the power of God and our Lady Mother the Virgin, in the name of the Father, Son and Holy Ghost. They used two to put it on you, I'll take it off you with three, with the power of God and the Virgin Mary. [C.7]

34 S. Ana had Jesus, saw him born, raised, baptized, anointed, blessed with the Sacraments. *Fulano*, what's the matter with you? *Olhado*, *quebrante*, who put it on you? It was an *olho mau*. They used two to put it on you, I'll take it off you with three, whether it came from an ugly man or a handsome one, at the time of your going out, when you were shopping, or paying, if it was caused by *mofina*, or *olho grosso*, or *olho mau*. It's not me taking it off but Jesus, Joseph and Mary. [S.1]

35 On my way from the olive groves to the mountains I met our Lord, he asked: —Where are you going? —I'm going to cure *olhado* Lord. He said —What do you cure with? —With your word, Lord, the eleven thousand virgins, the twelve apostles who accompanied you until you had died and risen again, Lord. Whether affecting the flesh, or the skin, or the nerves, or the blood, causing stitch or congestion, be gone to the waves of the holy sea where there is neither cock, nor hen, nor any cock crows. Ave Maria, ave Maria, ave Maria, they used two to put it on you, I'll use three to take it off you, with the power of God and the Virgin Mary. [C.6]

36 They used two to put it on you, I'll use three to take it off you, with the power of God and the Virgin Mary and the three persons of the Most Holy Trinity. *Olhado*, *quebrante*, *mofina*, and affliction of any parts which may be unknown to anybody, I cast out in the name of God, the Father Almighty, into the ebbing tide to where no cattle crow nor any hen, that no harm be done to any human being. I met S. Maça S. Maça and S. Marcelinho. I asked —With what do you pray? —With the name of God the Father, God the Son and God the Holy Ghost and the three persons of the Most Holy Trinity, *olhado*, *mofina* and all afflictions which may be unknown to anyone. Meeting Our Lady, her rosary in her hand, I asked for the rosary she said no, I asked again she gave me the string saying —no one can do anything with you, only the force of the three persons of the most Holy Trinity, Jesus, Mary, Joseph, the blessed chalice and the consecrated host, in the name of the Father, God the Son, God the Holy Ghost, may all evil forces you carry with you be removed, amen. If this *olhado*, this *mofina* came from your right hand side, I cast it out from the left, if from the left, I cast out from the right, if from behind, I cast out from the front, if from the front, I cast out from behind, in the name of God the Father, God the Son, God the Holy Ghost. [C.14]

The following prayer also invokes the assistance of the *caboclo* spirit

Paraguaçú, this being the only case I discovered in which the indigenous element has shown any influence on curing prayers.

37 *Fulano*, with two they overlooked you, with three I cure you, with the power of God and the Virgin. If they overlooked your eyes, hair, food, drink, clothes, progress of your life, with the power of God and the Virgin I remove this *quebrante*. The morning star, which announced the day, speak these good words to this brother curing this *olhado*, *mofina*, *quebrante*, putting them in the ebb tide where no cock crows, nor any hen, with the power of God and the Virgin Mary. *Caboclo* Paraguaçú I ask you with the powers God gave you, with your bow and arrows, influence [*encorrente*],[41] these evil spirits, these malingerers, be they ghosts or relatives, or if they were sent with the power of the Virgin Mary, I ask you to cleanse [*dar um passe*][42] and influence these evil ones. God the Father, God the Son and God the Holy Ghost. Amen. Our Lady of the Conception cover you with her mantle, may the divine Holy Spirit light your paths, praised be our Lord Jesus Christ for ever and ever. Amen.[43] [I.2]

Olhos (eyes)

Prayers for the eyes fall into four distinct categories. The first two reveal a sense of urgency and should be recited when something has become lodged unexpectedly in the eye. The reciter does not use herbs in this case, but lifts the eyelid between his thumb and forefinger and gently moves it with a circular motion:

38 S. Lucia passed this way, her little horse eating grass. I gave her bread, she said no, I gave her wine, she said yes.[44] [I.2]

39 Make haste, horseman, through São Pedro's door. Tell Santa Lucia to send me a white kerchief to remove this speck of dust.[45] [S.1]

The third type of prayer refers to Santa Lucia's three daughters:

40 Santa Lucia had three daughters, one sewed, one spun, and the other removed specks of dust from eyes.[46] [I.1]

The fourth category of prayer covers more lasting and serious eye conditions, such as cataracts:

41 S. Luzia, by day and by night show me your light from the arm of the Holy Cross. If that cloud contained water, or some kind of contaminated water, or if it was some kind of witchcraft, may this cloud be carried away into the sky, with the power of God and the Virgin Mary.[47] [C.3]

Parto (childbirth)

The mother shouts out the following prayer during the final stages of labour in order to be rid of the placenta:

42 Santa Margarida, I am neither pregnant nor delivered. Take this rotten flesh from my womb.[48] [I.2]

Another type of prayer, also said by the mother when in labour, requests that the baby should be born before the priest finishes saying mass.

43 Our Lady of the birth come and help me. The priest in the church is saying holy mass. Before the priest finishes this child will come. The Blessed Virgin Mary help me too, help this child to come so I can lay him in my hands. The Holy Spirit rose to speak to Jesus so that this mother in labour might rest.[49] [C.6]

Queimadura (burn)

The prayer mentions Santa Sofia and her three daughters, the last of whom is able to extinguish fire and overcome it:

44 Santa Sofia had three daughters. One spun, one sewed, and one quenched the flames of the fire.[50] [S.1]

Sol na cabeça (sunstroke)

A folded towel is placed over a glass full of water. Both towel and glass are then upturned and placed on top of the patient's head. As the water seeps away through the towel, bubbles begin to rise in the glass and this is believed to be the water boiling as it comes into contact with the heat of the sun in the head. After the prayer, the towel is shaken outside the door (I.2). This can be done at any time during the day.[51]

45 When God was in the world He caught much sun and heat. He met our Lady who told Him that the sun was got rid of with an eyecloth and a glass of cold water. As I speak the truth this woman returns the sun to its place beneath the sea with a little glass of cold water. The evil that is in his (her) body and head, remove it, God and the Virgin Mary. [I.2]

C.13, however, does not upturn the glass, but stands it the right way up on the patient's head. After reciting the following prayer, he makes a circle with the glass three times round the patient's head:

46 God is sun, God is light, God is clarity, and God is the three persons of the Holy Trinity. This headache, if it was sun or if it was night air.[52] [C.13]

Soluço (hiccups)

The patient says the following three times in one breath:

47 Hiccups go, hiccups come, hiccups go to someone else.[53]

Torcedura, *torção*, *torcido*, *desmentidura* (sprains, dislocations)

The ritual that most commonly accompanies the prayers consists of the reciter symbolically sewing with a needle and thread, and sometimes passing these through a piece of material held above the affected area (I.1, I.8, C.11).[54] I.2 passes a reel of cotton with a virgin needle fixed in it round and round the affected area. After the prayer, the reel and needle should be placed near the stove, and after being used for the last time, should be thrown into the ebbing tide.

48 What Frutuoso prays for, twisted nerves, torn flesh, dislocated bones, with the power of God and São Frutuoso this bone will return to its place, with the power of God and the Virgin Mary. Amen.[55] [I.2]

Another method consists of blessing the affected area with three pieces of clay taken from the wall of a house (S.1, C.13) while saying the following:

49 São Frutuoso. What does he pray for? Torn flesh, twisted nerves, broken veins, broken bones, with the power of God and the Virgin Mary. [S.1]

C.13's prayer mentions the act of sewing, despite the fact that he only accompanies it by blessing with the three pieces of clay:

50 I pray and I sew torn flesh, bruised flesh, twisted nerves, broken nerves, sprains, twisted nerves, praise be to Senhor Fortuoso. I pray just like this, I sew just like this, praise be to São Fortuoso. [C.13]

A further method involves a woman who has given birth to twins placing her foot (either left or right) on the sprain/dislocation.[56] If the patient is a man, the woman must be the mother of twin girls; if a woman, the twins should be boys. The mother of the twins should accompany her act with the following prayer:

51 You want me to pray for you, for a sprain, torn flesh, broken nerves, dislocated bones. [C.7]

Vento mal; ar, moléstia do ar (ill wind)

Vento mal covers all sudden deteriorations in health that cannot immediately be accounted for. To a certain extent, it is very similar in concept to *quebranto* in that it does not come as a result of an evil deliberately inflicted by one person on another. In fact, many of the symptoms for *vento mal* are similar and often identical to those associated with *quebranto* (for example, continual crying in infants; interrupted growth; general weakness; headaches; chills; sleeplessness),[57] and this accounts for the marked similarity between some of the prayers which mention *quebranto* and *vento mal* (or their synonyms) at the same time. The most serious illnesses caused by *vento mal* are coronary thrombosis, all forms of paralysis, other physical imperfections (such as speech defects) and mental disease.[58]

The *vento mal* is considered literally to be a wind that carries with it misfortunes that may strike anyone at any time.[59] Even a footprint can be *atingido pelo ar* ('touched by the *ar*') and everyone is at all times vulnerable (I.3). It is therefore greatly feared, and a great deal of care surrounds the recitation of prayers to counter it. C.6 places a clove of *alho macho* behind each ear and blesses each of her wrists with a third clove before commencing the prayer. S.1 makes the sign of the cross and recites the *Pater Noster* before the curing prayer so as to protect herself from any evil that might strike her on leaving the patient. Curing prayers for *vento mal* must never be recited on a Friday,[60] and it is always advisable to chew a clove of garlic during recitation (C.11, S.1). The patient should be blessed with herbs, first of all on the left-hand side and then on the right (C.6). Recitation should never take place at night (I.2), nor should it be accompanied by charcoal but always by freshly picked herbs (S.1). The patient should have broken his fast before the prayer is recited (S.5).

Two of the prayers collected list the possible origins of the *ar* that is making the patient ill:

52 São Romão was born in Rome. São Romão was baptized there. This wind which has entered your body, be it in your food, or your drink, or your rest, or your rising, or your bathing, or washing your feet, through space, through footprint, through the day, through the evening, through the night, through the noon, with the power of God and the Virgin Mary throw this wind in the sea, in the ebb tide. Amen. [C.13]

53 Maria take your lamp and go to the virgins' kingdom, born in Rome, baptized in Rome, conceived in Rome, died in Rome, buried in Rome, be it paralysis, *vento*, madness, *esquecido* [*sic*], *espramisido* [*sic*], deformity, *torino* [*sic*], lameness, get out, *vento mal*, away to the waves of the sacred sea with the power of God and the Virgin. [C.7]

Another embodies a conversation between the reciter and Jesus Christ:

54 Going to Jerusalem I met Jesus Christ. He asked me: —Where are you going? —Lord, I'm going to cure *moléstia do ar*. —What do you cure with? —With a branch, Lord. He said: It that all? —With garlic passed over the wrists, Lord, it's a dangerous disease but I'm not afraid, my Saviour. I cure with your blood, with your strength I drive out everything into the waves of the sacred sea or into the wind, just as Cipriano cured. [C.6]

The next prayer mentions cabbalistic numbers (3, 7, 14 and 21), and colours ranging from black to white. The transition from black to pure white is supposed to represent a transition from evil to good in that, as the colours become lighter, so the evil is rejected. (Colour symbolism of this nature is also employed in the ritual called *trabalho*. See below, page 124.)

55 Senhor S. Romão or Manuel or Maria saw the evil wind, and Jesus in Egypt replied: —Pray my son against this evil. He who was born in Egypt (and not created), dead and buried, go out of here *vento mau*. Go to the ebbing tide where no Christian passes, nor does the cock crow, nor the sheep caw.[61] I pray with three, with seven, with fourteen and twenty-one, from black, red, green and white. This evil will remain there never to return, in the name of our Lord, the three persons and the Virgin Mary. Glory to the Father and Son and to the Holy Ghost. [S.1]

The ill wind is also associated with minor mental disturbances in the recently bereaved. If the patient is constantly disturbed by seeing a dead relative or friend in dreams or in ghost form, he is believed to be suffering from *mofina* or *mofina de morto*, and the following prayer is recited:

56 São João baptized Christ, Christ baptized João. The two was baptized in the river Jordan. Spirit of the dead, shade of the dead, ghost of the dead, perturbing presence of the dead, evil eyes of the dead, *mofina* and *quebrante de morto*, go far away from this body. [C.13]

Ar de morto is another condition associated with the *vento mal* and is very much akin to *mofina*. However, in the case of *ar de morto*, the patient does not see the dead person in dreams or in ghost form. It is believed that the dead person's spirit lingers near the living and distracts them, and that if it is not driven away the living may become ill. The *ar de morto* is feared so much because of its association with the *egun* (spirits of the dead) who, when in possession of their mediums, constantly strive to mingle with the onlookers. It is believed that if an *egun* touches a living person, he brings death; and in Amoreiras (Itaparica) there is a constant fear of the *egun*, not because they are evil, but because they want to be reincarnated in the living. A common synonym for *ar de morto* is *egun*, as shown in the following prayer:

57 Holy and just body of God, by the blood of Christ so help me God. I beg by the five wounds of our Lord Jesus Christ, the first wound of his blessed head was made by a crown of thorns offending your temples, and your blood spilt and covered your face that it might wash away the sins of the world, your feet and hands was nailed to the cross. Your blessed heart was pierced with a lance and the wounding of the blessed

left shoulder was the most painful wound which Christ felt in his body. Take away this dead man's spirit, this *egun*, day, night, or noon. I am praying over you as Most Holy Mary prayed. She incensed her Blessed Son in order that he might smell sweet. I pray over your body that the evil may be cast out and the good enter in.[62] [I.8]

Ventre caído

There is no adequate equivalent in accepted scientific medical terminology for *ventre caído*, but it is clear that the illness is very closely linked to the notion that sufferers have been struck by the evil eye in that many of the symptoms are similar. It only ever occurs in children who are particularly exposed to the dangers of the evil eye, and symptoms are usually restlessness, sleeplessness and prolonged crying.[63]

A common means of diagnosis consists of measuring the infant's feet one against the other to see if there is any discrepancy. If they are not equal, the infant is considered to be suffering from *ventre caído* (I.2 and *passim*). This is similar to the method of diagnosing *espinhela caída*, already described above (page 97), and may derive from the same source. It is also linked to the idea that overlooking (*quebranto*) causes stunted growth as described above (page 76).

The prayer should be recited over and over again while the reciter makes a cross with his thumb on the following parts of the infant's body: left palm, left elbow, right elbow, chest, navel, both knees held together, both sides of the feet held together (I.2).[64] The baby may then be lifted up into the air by the feet three times and the feet are made to touch the door lock or the lintel (C.7). The baby is then turned on its back, and crosses again are made on the following parts of its body: back, buttocks, back of the knees pushed together, soles of the feet pushed together. It may now be lifted again to touch the lock or the lintel.[65]

58 Doors open facing the sea. *Ventre caído* find your rightful place. With the keys of the sanctuary I will raise your *ventre*, with the power of God and the Virgin Mary. [C.13]

Another prayer associates the cure of *ventre caído* with the birth, death and resurrection of Christ:

59 God was born, God died, God rose again. He raised up *ventre caído* with the power of God and the Virgin Mary. Amen.[66] [I.2]

Verruga (wart)

It is commonly believed that warts originate from pointing at stars or at the moon (I.2 and *passim*), and according to some, the number of warts acquired is equal to the number of stars that are pointed at (I.1, C.7, S.1).[67] A cure consists of pointing a sharp knife at a very bright star or at the moon and saying:

60 Star, moon, my wart said you must die and it must live. [I.2 and *passim*]

The knife is then pointed at the wart and made to touch it (C.6 blesses the wart with the knife) saying:

But I say that you must live and it must die.[68]

*

There are certain aspects of these prayers which are worthy of note. On the whole, they are based on European tradition and show little tendency to embrace influences from African and indigenous cultures, the main exception here being No. 37 (page 103) in which the *caboclo* spirit Paraguaçú is invoked to assist in curing the evil eye, and No. 57 (page 108–9) which contains a brief reference to an *egun*. Other differences are purely linguistic and are based on changes being made in the words of the prayer in order to adapt to Brazilian usage. Hence, for example, prayers for *erisipela* from Portugal contain the use of the Portuguese *tornar* (to return), whereas in Brazil the verb *tornar* tends to be found less commonly than *voltar* in the original Portuguese transcriptions.

In one example, however, the language has not surrendered fully to Portuguese and continues to show slight Spanish (Galician?) influence, perhaps betraying the possible Portugal/Spain border origins of the original prayer. I refer to No. 31 (page 101), which in the original reads the Spanish *Padre* (Father) in the last phrase and not the Portuguese *Pai*.

The peculiarly oral nature of the curing prayer has led to slight corruption of certain words which in fact change the meaning of the sentence completely. Hence Gouveia (1926:27) gives a prayer for *engasgo* which calls São Braz the *escrivão* (scribe) of Christ, while prayer No.14 (page 94) refers to him as being Christ's *escravo* (slave). Similarly, prayer No. 36 (page 102) (for the evil eye) refers to sending away the evil with the ebbing tide: '... to where no cattle crow'. The original *gado* (cattle) here should, in fact, be *galo* (cockerel) to balance *galinha* (hen). All other versions encountered give *galo* instead of *gado*, the only exception being Nunes (1950:46).

Some words in the prayers are unidentifiable in standard dictionaries, though to the person reciting the prayer they have a most specific meaning. Hence, in prayer No. 10 (page 93) (*dor de cabeça*), *chaqueta* and *maleta* refer to different types of pain that may be experienced when suffering from a headache. In prayer No. 53 (page 107) (*vento*), *espramisido* and *torino* are meaningless and could not be explained by the informant. *Esquecido* (forgotten) is included in the same prayer, but has little meaning in the context unless it is to be read as meaning loss of memory. In prayer No. 55 (page 108) (*vento*), *gorgoveia* is also meaningless, first because it is a corruption of *corveja* (third person singular of *corvejar* = to caw, crow), and secondly because the verb *balir* (to bleat) should have been used in the context.

Mar sagrado (sacred sea), which appears in many of the prayers, may in fact be a corrupt version of *mar salgado* (salty sea),[69] and in the following prayer for the evil eye, given by Valle (1962:598), salt and the sacred sea are linked:

Just as this salt was created in the sacred sea may it be good enough to take away this *quebranto* or *mau olhado* put on by dead or living or by an excommunicated devil.

Another feature of the oral style is that Saints Peter and Paul, who appear in many of the prayers, are looked upon as being one person. The verb governing them in the original Portuguese is almost always in the singular, and they are referred to as *Pedro Paulo* and not *Pedro e Paulo* (Peter and Paul).[70] This tendency for plural subjects to be governed by a verb in the singular is quite common, e.g. No. 56 (page 108), 'The two was baptized' (orig. *Todos dois foi batizado*), and No. 57: '... your feet and hands was nailed to the cross' (orig. *foi cravados os vossos pés na cruz e as vossas mãos*).

One very noticeable characteristic of many of the prayers is their close link with the science of astrology. There are many references, both in the wording of the prayer and in the instructions that accompany it, to different heavenly bodies and their movements in the sky. This is probably based on the medieval notion that movements of the cosmos could bring sickness, and thus, in the same way, similar movements could bring about a cure.[71] Hence warts may disappear with the cycle of the moon, as shown in the following prayer transcribed by Braun (1950:57):

God bless you, new moon which I see before me now. By the next moon the warts will have gone.

or by entreating a star or the moon to destroy the wart as shown in prayer No. 60 (page 110). Toothache is also dispatched in the name of the rising sun and setting moon (e.g. prayer No. 12, page 94) and it is considered important to recite prayers for curing *espinhela caída* and *ventre caído* at daybreak so that, as the sun rises to its highest position in the sky, it may assist in raising the so-called 'fallen' matter back to its former position (I.2 and *passim*). The frequent references to sending away illness and all forms of evil (*mau olhado*, *vento*) with the ebbing tide is another reflection of the importance attached to the phase of the moon at a given time (see especially prayers Nos. 20, 36, 37 and 55, pages 96, 102, 103 and 108 respectively).

CHAPTER XI

EBÓ

Various definitions have been given of the term *ebó*. It means principally 'sacrifice' or 'offering', and the term *despachar ebó* means to undertake a sacrifice of some kind with a view to ridding oneself of evil or a certain influence that may be making one ill.[1] The object that is to be sacrificed must first of all be rubbed against the body in such a way that any evil or undesirable influence may pass from the body into the object. The object must then be left in a suitable place where the evil in it can dissipate without doing any harm to others. Such places are usually a crossroads, the sea at ebb tide, a river, sewer outlet or entrance to a cemetery. The objects, once used, are also referred to by the term *ebó*.[2]

An individual may undertake an *ebó* on himself. This type of *ebó* will be termed 'simple' *ebó*. It is usually a very simple ceremony that takes place with no onlookers or assistants, on a beach at the ebb tide, on the banks of a river, or simply facing the setting sun. The individual concerned rubs the objects he has brought over his body, starting from the torso and proceeding along the length of each limb. The object is then cast into the water or buried directly in line with the setting sun. Objects may vary from a candle to cigars, *acaçá*,[3] bananas, chocolate and cakes. Just as it is important to leave the objects in a place where they can do no harm to others, so it is considered extremely propitious to undertake such a ritual at the end of the calendar year, so that any undesirable influence affecting the individual concerned may disappear with the old year. This is particularly the case in the south of Brazil, especially in Rio de Janeiro, where cult followers may be seen in their thousands making such offerings on Copacabana beach on the night of 31 December.[4] Sometimes the individual stands knee-deep in the sea and pours over his head bottles of *cachaça*, wine or champagne.

The simplest form of *ebó* involves no sacrifice as such, but merely a symbolic cleaning of the body. The individual wipes his hands over his torso, shoulders, back and legs, and finally along his arms towards the wrists, which should be held out in the direction of the sea. This simple ceremony is described as *limpar-se* (to cleanse oneself).

The types of *ebó* described so far involve the participation only of the individual concerned, who may undergo this ritual either as a preventive measure to ensure that all undesirable forces are kept away, or because he feels that his body should be cleansed of a specific force of evil that may be responsible for making him ill. He may contribute to the overall effect of the *ebó* by taking a ritual bath, fumigating himself, applying *pemba*, or he might also arrange to have a *sacudida*. However, if the illness in question is such that it does not respond to any of this treatment, the individual involved may have to arrange to undergo a considerably more complex *ebó* known also as *trabalho* (work) or *limpeza de corpo* (cleansing of the body).

The main difference between a 'simple' and 'complex' *ebó* is that the latter is always presided over and conducted by a *pai* or *mãe de santo*, and it is this presence of someone in authority that makes the 'complex' *ebó* an extremely powerful instrument with which to bring about a cure. The entire ritual, though basically similar to the simple *ebó*, is conducted on a considerably higher and more formal level. The officiating *pai* or *mãe* is dressed in ritual clothing, and he wears the beads of office (*contas*) which are believed to form an extremely close link between the wearer and the *orixás* they represent.[5] The ritual is accompanied by incantations and prayers that exhort the *orixás* to assist in bringing about a successful cure.

From the very beginning, the *orixás* play a leading role in the *trabalho*, in that it is the *orixá* of the *pai* or *mãe de santo* in question who decides whether or not a patient should undergo a *trabalho*. Every *trabalho* is preceded by a *consulta* (consultation) that takes place between the patient and the *orixá* of his *pai* or *mãe de santo*. This means that the *pai* or *mãe* falls into a trance and assumes the identity of the *orixá* to whom he or she belongs. This *orixá* then speaks through the medium of the *pai* or *mãe* to the patient and informs him of the reason for his illness and gives him advice as to what precise action should be taken in order to overcome it.

The illness may turn out to be caused by one of three main factors:

1. *Queda de orixá:* this term means literally 'fall of (the) *orixá*', and it refers to the moment when a person is possessed by his *orixá* for the first time.[6] This generally takes place in a cult house during a festival, and the *orixá* concerned is usually the same as the *orixá* whose drum rhythm and incantations are at the time being played and sung. The person, once possessed, is taken directly to the *camarinha* (small room) and starts his initiation from that moment (C.12). However, *queda de orixá* is an elastic term also used to refer to certain other indications,

sent by the *orixá* to the person concerned, that he should become initiated into the cult. These may vary from minor indispositions, such as headaches or bouts of nausea, to major illnesses, such as smallpox (I.2).

Sometimes the *queda de orixá* may be looked upon as being the reason for a number of misfortunes which would cease immediately if the person concerned became initiated into the cult. I.1 had lost two children within eighteen months of each other in household accidents and laid the blame entirely on the fact that her *orixá* (Yansan) was angry at her not becoming initiated into the cult. Similar stories were told by I.8 and C.14.

Illness may also be sent by an *orixá* to a person already initiated into the cult who has not kept up his ritual obligations. The illness in this case may be cured by some form of ritual offering, again dictated by the *orixá* of the *pai* or *mãe de santo* consulted. The offering may vary from a dish of food left in the *pejí* to the sacrifice of one or more of the animals that come under the control of the offended *orixá* (C.2).[7]

2. The spirit of a dead relative or friend who remains near the living and torments them in such a way that they become ill. Such a spirit is often called an *egun*. It must be stressed, however, that an *egun* is not considered to be in any way evil, but rather just an undesirable factor that may endanger the well-being of the living.

3. The presence inside the body of an evil spirit that stops it functioning in the correct way. Such an evil spirit may be called *um exú* ('an exú'), although, as has been pointed out before, Exú the *orixá* is not by nature evil.

If, during the consultation, the *orixá* identifies the patient's illness as stemming from *queda de orixá*, he will advise that the only method of cure is initiation into the cult. The cure would then come about as the various initiatory rituals are performed. If the illness stems from neglect of ritual obligations, then the *orixá* consulted will dictate the precise nature of the sacrifices or offerings that should be made to appease the anger of the individual's *orixá*.

In the case of 2 and 3, however, the *orixá* consulted would advise that the patient should undergo a *trabalho* or *limpeza de corpo*. At the same time, the *orixá* gives precise details as to which specific ingredients should be employed, together with the exact quantities of each. Sometimes the *orixá* himself writes out the list of articles required as an *aide-mémoire* for the patient (I.2, I.4, I.5, C.2). C.6, on the other hand, mentioned that certain articles (for example, the number of candles employed during the ritual) are standard, and the *orixá* rarely modifies the number required. When the *pai* or *mãe de santo* comes out of the trance, the patient informs him or her of the result of the *consulta*[8] and must then begin to gather together all the articles required. This may take months. In one *trabalho* witnessed, the patient, who was particularly poor, had been saving the money for her *trabalho* for eighteen months.

The cost varies according to the size of *trabalho* prescribed by the *orixá*, but in addition to the actual cost of the ingredients, the patient must also pay the *pai* or *mãe de santo* for his services, and meet the cost of what is known as *dinheiro do chão* (floor money). The cost of the *pai* or *mãe de santo*'s services is fixed according to the social standing of the patient, but it is never below Cr$200.00, and may go as high as Cr$4,000.00.[9] This is paid before the ritual begins. The *dinheiro do chão* is the payment made by the patient to the *carregador do ebó* (carrier of the *ebó*), who is a man (rarely a woman) appointed by the *pai* or *mãe de santo* to take all the ingredients after the ritual and deposit them in a suitable place. Although the *dinheiro do chão* is a payment made by the patient, it must be handed over to the *carregador do ebó* not by the patient but by the *pai* or *mãe de santo*. Moreover, it cannot form part of the payment made to the *pai* or *mãe* for acting during the ritual. It must be in a separate package and should be handed to the *pai* or *mãe* well before the ritual starts, and if possible the day before. Again, the *dinheiro do chão* varies according to the size of the *trabalho* and the social standing of the patient, but in the *trabalhos* witnessed (I.2, C.2), the *dinheiro do chão* amounted to approximately a quarter of the payment made to the *mãe* or *pai*. The *dinheiro do chão* is either left literally on the floor, where it can be easily picked up by the *carregador* at the end of the ritual, or placed inside a small box on which the patient sits (C.6).[10] Alternatives are to leave the money underneath the patient's left foot (I.2), or for the *pai* or *mãe* to give it to the *carregador* before the ritual begins (C.2).[11]

A *trabalho* designed specifically to rid the patient of an *egun* is known as *trabalho* (or *limpeza*) *para discarrego de um egun*. As mentioned above (page 51 n. 17), the word *discarrego* should in fact be *descarregamento*, meaning 'unburdening'. Hence the full translation would be: *trabalho/limpeza* to unburden (a patient) of an *egun*.

The following ritual was not witnessed, since the patient requested that it should be conducted in total secrecy. It was, however, described to me afterwards by C.6, the *mãe de santo* who officiated. The ritual was accompanied by incantations, but C.6 was not able to ascertain precisely what had been sung since she had conducted most of the ritual in a trance.

The ingredients in order of use were as follows:

green cabbage leaves
mustard plant leaves
okra (in one of the following quantities: 3, 7, 14 or 21)
500 grams capsicums
500 grams tomatoes
500 grams manioc flour mixed with olive or vegetable oil
500 grams maize
500 grams popcorn
9 *acaçá* (some red, some white)
1 live pigeon or dove

The patient sits on a small box which contains the *dinheiro do chão*. The *mãe de santo* makes a small cross on the patient's forehead with white solid *pemba*, and then draws three crossed swords on the floor behind the patient as in Figure 3. The design of sword hilt is that of Yansan, who alone among all the *orixás* in the myths was able to withstand the *egun* (see above, page 15).[12] All the ingredients are placed on plates on the floor around the patient, except the *acaçá*, which are left to one side. The *mãe* then picks up handfuls of each substance in the order given above, and makes as if to wipe the substance over the patient's body. In fact, she

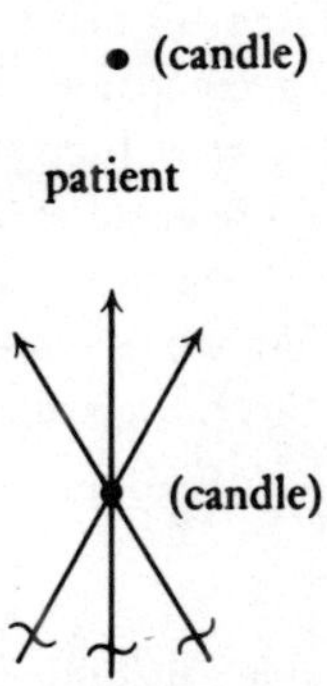

FIGURE 3.

never touches the patient, but working down from the head to the feet, allows each handful to drop on to the floor. The pigeon or dove is always the last item to be passed over the patient, but this should be done with extreme care so as not to injure it. The *carregador do ebó* places all the ingredients in an earthenware bowl known as an *alguidar*, and takes them together with the pigeon and the *acaçá* to a crossroads. The *alguidar* is left on the side of the road at the crossroads, and the pigeon, clearly a representation of the spirit that has been tormenting the patient, is set at liberty, and allowed to fly away.[13] The *carregador do ebó* then returns to the scene of the ritual, wiping the *acaçá* over his own body as he returns. He should return by a different route and not look behind him. He takes these precautions so that none of the undesirable forces should affect him.

Directly after the *trabalho*, the patient takes an *abó* and is then fumigated by the *mãe* with a mixture of incense and various herbs that attract forces of good. The patient must observe certain taboos, such as remaining *de corpo limpo* for at least three days and refraining from eating any of the ingredients used in the *trabalho* for a similar period.

A *trabalho* designed specifically to rid the patient of an Exú is known as *trabalho* (or *limpeza*) *para discarrego de um Exú* (*trabalho/limpeza* to unburden (a patient) of an Exú).[14] Because Exú is immediately associated with evil, various rituals must precede the *trabalho* so as to ensure success. In this sense, a *trabalho* to rid the body of an Exú is somewhat more complicated than the one just described, which rids the body of an *egun*. First, the *pai* or *mãe de santo* must conduct the ritual known as *o despacho da porta* (for description, see above, page 67). This is followed by fumigation of the premises, starting with substances to repel forces of evil, and continuing with substances designed to attract forces of good. This fumigation ceremony is accompanied by incantations (given above, pages 45–6). Each person present is fumigated individually, the censer on both occasions being passed beneath each armpit.

Two *trabalhos* of this nature were witnessed, and a third was described after the event, again by C.6. Trabalhos A and C involved just one patient, while Trabalho B involved three. Ingredients in order of use were as follows:

Trabalho A

1 dish full of mixed raw vegetables (including cooking bananas, capsicums, tomatoes, aubergines) chopped up

1 rag doll and needle and cotton
cigars (in one of the following quantities: 3, 5, 7, 9, 14, 21)
approx. 1 square metre each of plain black, red and white cloth
500 grams black beans
500 grams 'garlic' maize (*milho de alho*)
500 grams white beans
500 grams popcorn
500 grams white maize (*milho branco*) cooked
5 *acaçá*
1 live cockerel, preferably dark in colour
2 reels white cotton
gunpowder
[I.2]

Trabalho B

3 reels white cotton
manioc flour mixed with *dendê* oil/*cachaça*/water
7 large okra
3 raw eggs
approx. 1 square metre each of plain black, red and white cloth
7 cigars
1 kilo toasted maize (*milho torrado*)
7 *acaçá* (red and white)
3 banana leaves }
3 sprigs *vassourinha de Nossa Senhora* } for *sacudida*
7 sprigs *coerana* }
1 cockerel (colour not important)
gunpowder
[C.2]

Trabalho C

3 cotton reels (black, red, white)
manioc flour mixed with *dendê* oil/*cachaça*/ water
1 bottle *cachaça*
7 cigars
1 litre black beans

1 litre manioc flour
1 litre 'garlic' maize (*milho de alho*)
1 kilo maize flour
1 kilo rice
1 kilo popcorn
1 cockerel, preferably black or red and black
[C.6]

In each case, certain cabbalistic signs were drawn on the floor with *pemba*. The sign for Trabalho C was identical to that given above (page 117), and those for the other two were as in Figures 4 and 5. C.2 mentioned how the sign he chooses varies with each *trabalho* he performs, though he always uses the same three colours (white, green, red) and a combination of the pentangle, circle and arrow-like design reproduced in Figure 5.

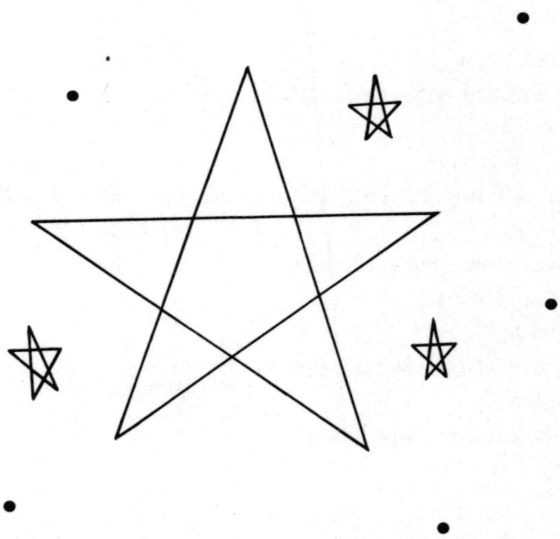

FIGURE 4. Cabbalistic sign for Trabalho A (I.2).

The different coloured *pembas* used in Figure 5 are significant in that green is the colour of Oxossi, who is the *orixá* who controls the *pai de santo* in question. The *pai* always includes Oxossi's colour in *trabalhos* of this nature, since he feels it is his duty to invoke the assistance of his *orixá* before all others. Red is the colour of Yansan who is considered by this particular *pai* to be very efficacious in driving away not just an *egun*

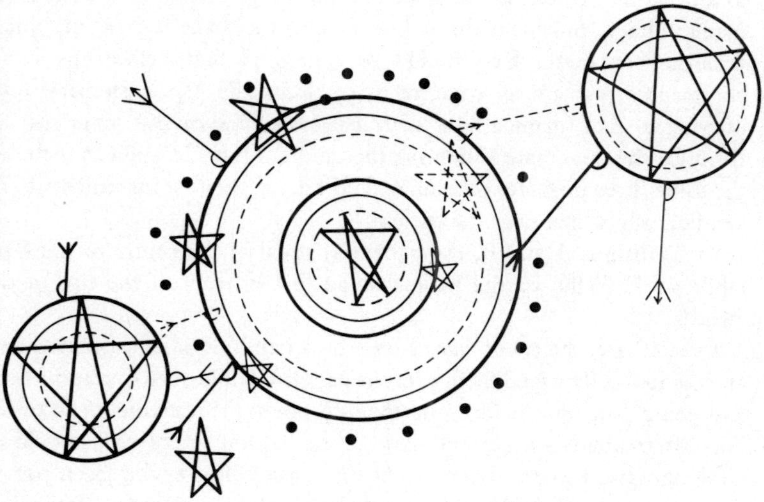

[— = white *pemba*] [-- = red *pemba*]
[— = green *pemba*] [• = candle]

FIGURE 5. Cabbalistic sign for Trabalho B (C. 2).

but also an Exú. In fact, we shall see in the transcribed prayers below (see especially No. 1 (page 126) and No. 29 (page 130) that the terms are confused and that the *egun* and Exú are given virtually the same identity. A similar confusion is made by C.6, who uses the same sign (the three crossed swords of Yansan) to drive away both the *egun* and Exú. All three informants (I.2, C.2 and C.6) were able to distinguish between *egun* and Exú, the main criterion being that the former is not considered to be by nature malicious, but I.2 and C.2 admitted that they follow precisely the same ritual in both cases. C.6, however, conducted separate, albeit similar, rituals, despite the identical chalked sign in each case.[15]

In all cases, candles were set up and lit all round the patient(s), one being placed outside the *pejí* or house in honour of Exú (the *orixá* as opposed to the evil spirit), while all the others were placed round the signs on the floor, as shown in the illustrations. In the case of Trabalho C, the candles numbered eight as opposed to two in the *trabalho para discarrego de um egun* already described (see page 117 above), the additional six being positioned in a circle around the sign and the patient. The candle given to Exú should be the first withdrawn from the packet, and should be lit and positioned outside before any other preparations for the ritual are made. This is linked to the notion behind the *pade de Exú*, in which, according to myth, Exú should be honoured first before any ritual commences (see above, page 32 n. 5). I.2 made the customary food offering to Exú (manioc flour with *dendê* oil, *cachaça* and water respectively) at the same time as lighting the candle, while C.2 and C.6 included the same three mixtures of manioc flour among the first ingredients to be symbolically wiped over the patient.

In Trabalhos A and B, the patient(s) stood in the centre of the sign, while in Trabalho C, the patient stood just in front of the tips of the swords.

In each case, the *pai* or *mãe de santo* took handfuls of all the ingredients and symbolically wiped them over the patients' bodies, starting at the head and going down to the feet, and then dropping the ingredients on to the floor. Ingredients such as the okra, cigars, cotton reels (see also below), cloth and *acaçá* were broken or cut into pieces after having been passed over the patient's body, thus symbolizing the destruction of the evil spirit. The rag doll in Trabalho A was trampled beneath the patient's left foot and then torn in two pieces. Even the candles gathered up at the end of the *trabalho* were broken before being included with the rest of the ingredients and taken away by the *carregador do ebó*.

All three cases included the use of cotton reels. C.6 employed three reels of different colours at the very beginning to test if the *trabalho* could be performed successfully. The patient stood with legs apart, and the *mãe* bent down in front of her and handed the thread of each reel through the patient's legs to her assistant standing behind the patient. The assistant then pulled all the threads at the same time, while the *mãe* allowed the reels to unwind in her hands. It was believed that if the black thread turned out to be longer than the other two, then the *trabalho* should be put off until another day.

C.2, at the very beginning of the ritual, wound three entire cotton reels (white) round the bodies of the three patients, and at the end of the ritual cut the cotton away, thus symbolically cutting away the evil influence that had made them ill. I.2's method was similar, in that she first symbolically wiped the three white cotton reels over the patient's body and then unwound each reel, breaking the thread at intervals.

Each case included the use of a cockerel as a scapegoat. The patient held it in such a way as to be able to approach the cock's beak to his mouth. The patient then spoke very softly to the cockerel, telling it to take away all the harmful forces of evil and to leave his body free of illness. After this, the *pai* or *mãe* symbolically wiped the cockerel over the patient's body and then proceeded to sacrifice it. The patient and all the onlookers had to turn their backs on the scene. Each wing and leg were washed and then broken before the cockerel was killed, either by cutting with a knife just below the beak (I.2, C.2) or by pushing the knife forwards through a freshly picked *folha da Costa*. A cockerel sacrificed with a backwards thrust of the knife would not be accepted by Exú (C.6). C.2 specified that the knife should be brand new and subsequently taken away with the other ingredients.

I.2 and C.2 both mentioned that sacrifice of the cockerel would still take place even if the *trabalho* was being conducted for the specific purpose of driving away an *egun*, while C.6 saw the element of sacrifice as being the main difference between the two types of *trabalho* (and it should be noted how the pigeon in the ritual conducted by C.6 was not sacrificed). C.6 remarked: *O egun não deve beber sangue—é perigoso* ('The *egun* must not drink blood—it is dangerous'). Her insistence on this point is another example of the way *Candomblé de caboclo* differs at times quite radically from traditional practices. Cockerels, hens and on occasion goats are sacrificed and then cooked just before *egun* festivals (all of which is traditional practice) on the island of Itaparica, to ensure that the *egun*, when in possession of their mediums, may eat. On one occasion observed, the *egun* in question refused to give advice to an inquirer until a cockerel had been sacrificed in proper ritual fashion. Lima (1946:82) recounts how one cockerel was killed actually by an *egun*:

Apareceu sob a forma duma nebulosa, por vêzes se confundindo com as árvores, e, ao chegar ao local em que se encontrava o galo destinado à matança, foi diminuindo de volume até cair sôbre a ave indefesa, ouvindo-se apenas o grito do galo que morria. E do mesmo modo como havia chegado, desapareceu. Neste galo, ninguém mais toca. [Quoted by Bastide 1961:172]

(It [the *egun*] appeared in the form of a cloud, at times blending with the trees, and when it arrived at the place where the cockerel that was to be sacrificed was standing, it got smaller and smaller and then fell upon the helpless bird that gave out a weak cry as it died. And then it left in the same way as it had arrived. Nobody touched the cockerel from that moment on.)

Pieces of plain black, red and white cloth were symbolically wiped over the patient in Trabalhos A and B. After use each piece, with the exception of the white, which was left intact, was held above the patient's head and torn into strips. Informants I.2 and C.2 both pointed out the apparent colour symbolism here, in that the colour black was supposed to attract to it the majority of the evil influence in the patient's body with red attracting the remainder. White represented the ensuing pure state of the body. Neither informant associated the colour red in this instance with Yansan.

There is a certain amount of colour symbolism also in the order in which the different foods are passed over the body. The darker-coloured foods tend to be used first, followed by the lighter ones, the change in the patient's state that is taking place being represented by a gradual change in the colour of the ingredients being used.

The transformation in the patient is also symbolized by first using raw ingredients to wipe over the patient's body, followed by cooked ingredients. Hence popcorn, white maize and toasted maize and the *acaçá* are left till all the other edible raw ingredients have been used. Sometimes this criterion is linked to that of colour, when the red *acaçá* should be used before the white, because it is cooked and is a deeper colour than the white *acaçá*.

Gunpowder was employed on all three occasions. I.2 placed small heaps around the patient, C.2 laid a continuous line of gunpowder all around the three patients and C.6 sprinkled gunpowder along the outline of the sign drawn on the floor and clapped three times, saying:

Pemba[16] is only sprinkled by those who know how. Only those who know how hunt in the bush. Exú *é*, Exú *é*, Exú *é*.[17]

A *sacudida* with herbs (*vassourinha de Nossa Senhora*, *banana* and *coerana*) took place in only one of the *trabalhos* witnessed (B), and after use each sprig was broken in three places and included with all the other ingredients that were later taken away.

In Trabalhos A, B and C, the patient was made to take an *abó* bath at the very end of the ceremony. I.2 insisted that the patient should run from the room where the *trabalho* had taken place without looking back. While the patients bathed, the *carregador* came and took away all the ingredients employed during the ritual. On returning from the *abó*, the patients were fumigated, first with substances to repel all evil, and then with other substances designed to attract forces of good. *Pemba* was then applied.

I.2 and C.2 accompanied the entire ritual with the prayers and incantations transcribed below. C.6 however, was again unable to supply this information as she had conducted most of the ritual in a trance.

Brief indication is made of the stage the ritual had reached at the time of each transcription.

Trabalho A (*I.2*)

1 Mixed vegetables, rag doll, cigars:

*Sacolé sacolé gim gim**.

2 Cloth, black beans, 'garlic' maize:

*Sacuendecuá sacuendecué**.

3 White beans, popcorn, white maize, *acaçá*:

*Sacanené taté**.

4 Cotton reel:

Father of Rome, Ogun the lacemaker, what has he [i.e. Exú] come to do here? Three stayed there and four came shouting,[18] *xé truá*, *xé truá*, *xé truá*.*

5 Fumigation:

Thanks be to God, oh my God, Praise be to God, oh my God, Blessed be the hour, oh my God, in which Ogun was born, oh my God.

This incantation is then repeated with the name of another *orixá* substituting Ogun on each occasion. The last verse goes as follows:

Blessed be the hour, oh my God, in which all the *orixás* were born, oh my God.

6 Fumigation:

Blessed be the valley, the valley, Mary, blessed be the valley, the valley, Mary, *oyu pé pé pé*, *oyu pé pé pá*, *oyu pé pé pé**, the *caboclo* Maiongá.[19]

7 End of ritual:

Blessed be our Lord Jesus Christ. Blessed be our Lord Jesus Christ. The peace of God be with all.

Trabalho B (*C*.2)

1 Opening prayer before commencement of ritual:

Open the ways of all those who are in need of charity, and may the doors of goodness be open to all, and Luanda, may the current of the stars, the current of the waters, and the current of the virgin jungle[20] pass through these children that they might be rid of all persecutions, witchcraft, sorcery, evil-doing, phantoms, let all these be swept away in the current of the Jordan. In the name of Almighty God, in the name of the glorious S. Antonio, Oxalá, Obaluayé, Ogun Pati-Curi[21] with all his phalanx, let these children be surrounded in the name of Almighty God. So be it. In the name of Almighty God, in the name of the phalanxes of the divine Holy Spirit, in the name of the currents of *Umbanda* and Luanda, I cut and anull all persecutions, phantoms, witchcraft, sorcery, evil-doing, be it by an Exú, or an *egun*, I encircle and expel from these bodies and loose them in Jordan's current. In the name of Almighty God, I beg the current of the stars to shelter these children of Oxalá, of Obaluayé, Ogun Pati-Curi and all his phalanx, *caboclo* Boiadeiro, *caboclo* Jurema, guardian of phantoms, *caboclo* Sultão das Matas,[22] guardian of all phantoms, and to carry away in Jordan's current all that may be in the bodies of these children. In the name of Almighty God, so be it.

2 The *pai* lays hands on patients' heads:

Abaluayé *atoto* my father Abaluayé help, my father Abaluayé is a *babalorixá*.[23]

The *pai* then shouts:

Atoto, Babá,[24] *atoto*, Babá.

3 Meet an old man on the road and take his blessing, God's blessing, Abaluayé give me your permission.

4 Babá[25] has arrived. Baobinaó[26] has arrived now. Father Baobinaó has arrived.

5 Oh Papa Abaluayé. I beg by your crown, I beg by the love for God, that you leave not your children in vain.

The *pai* then shouts:

Atoto, Babá.

6 Why call Abaluayé *chereguedé**? Oh my father Abaluayé *chereguedé*. Oh my grandfather Abaluayé *chereguedé*. Oh my godfather Obaluayé *chereguedé*. Oh my brother Obaluayé *chereguedé*. Oh my uncle Obaluayé *chereguedé*.

7 Long live Obaluayé, *tatá*,* from the waves of the sea, *tatá*, he's come to pull up a root, *tatá*, to cure his children, *tatá*.

8 Long live Obaluayé the *caboclo*.[27] Whoever meddles with him ends up mad.

The *pai* then shouts:

Atoto Babá.

9 Cotton is wrapped around the patients:

Omolú *kebelujá*, *kwelê kwelê jombalá* (*bis*), Omolú *kebelujá**

10 Cut away all obstacles,[28] breaking down all the forces of witchcraft and sorcery, evil-doing, with the power of the Holy Spirit, Abaluayé cutting, setting apart and anulling all the forces of evil which must be cut

out of the bodies of these children that good may surround them. My father Abaluayé, Oxalá and Nanan Buru[29] of the sacred sea, let us cut away all obstacles.

11 Manioc flour with *dendê*, *cachaça* and water:

E Ogun é *é tatá que malembé* é Ogun é *é tatá que malembé**.

12 Senhor Ogun, Senhor Ogun, Senhor Ogun is king of the sea. *Caboclo* Sete Estrelas[30] is here, but he's come to work.

13 Senhor Ogun, Senhor Ogun, Senhor Ogun's never failed. Senhor Ogun is a blessed son, blessed by Jesus.

14 Senhor Ogun, Senhor Ogun, Senhor Ogun's never failed. Senhor Ogun is one of the first who arrived in this village.[31] I, Ogun the warrior, am not one to deny my origins; I'm a son of the clear waters, and grandson of Yemanjá.

15 Your paths were opened by Ogun and Old Abaluayé. Your happiness will come with Ogun the warrior, with Boiadeiro, with Oxalá.

16 Ogun *goró gosí* give me *na jó*.* I ask Olorun give me *na jó*.

17 Okra:

He is the king of the stars. He works with São Jeromi. With a thunderclap he calls Xangô *locoyá* [or] Xangô *muí*.*

18 My Santa Bárbara with your beautiful crowns, for the love of God, Santa Bárbara, do not abandon your children. *Epa hei kawó Xangôka-biyesi le*.[32]

19 Cloth:

Oxalá is the father of Luanda, father of mercy of Luanda.

20 My father Oxalá help me to work. Oxalá is king of heaven, king of the earth, and king of the sea.

21 Look at the mango leaf Oxalá, look how the wind carries it to the sea, but look at me Oxalá, if my *caboclo* goes away I'll go in search.

22 Cigars:

Hail Naná, hail, hail to the greatness of Obaluayé, Obaluayé, Obalorixá, hail to the greatness of Old Oxalá.

23 It belongs to Naná, *euá euá euá eué**.

24 Mother Naná is the mother of the whole world. Mother Naná is mother of all the world.

25 Cutting cotton:

I ask the twenty-one *orixás* to work for these daughters, to annul all kinds of persecution, sorcery and witchcraft. I cut and annul with the force of the divine Holy Spirit to leave these bodies clean as the Virgin Mary cleansed the body of her Blessed Son. I'm going to cleanse these bodies removing all evil, all maleficent phantoms, all evils blocking their paths, I cut and annul all this, in the name of Almighty God. May Oxalá take care of these daughters Naná, in the name of God, Oxossi, the whole current of the stars and of the waters, the current of the virgin jungle, the current of Obaluayé, the current of Oxossi, and Yansan, removing from your body all sorcery, and evil, in the name of Oxalá, Ogun, Obaluayé and Naná Buruku, in the waves of the sacred sea. And Jordan's current will sweep away all the evil that may be in the bodies of these children. In the name of Almighty God. So be it. Oxalá grant me peace.

26 Who tied you up must also untie you.

27 I came for an *ebó* according to Nanan's orders. The work was done well for the girl to have an *ebó*. She is not having an *ebó*. No *ebó* is needed for she has Obaluayé[33] to succour her.

28 Gunpowder and *sacudida:*

The star of the sea is far out on the horizon. Let us send this *egun* out as well. The star of the sea is far out on the horizon. Let us send this Exú out as well. The star of the sea is far out on the horizon. Let us send this suffering out as well. The star of the sea is far out on the horizon. Let us send this persecution out as well. The star of the sea is far out on the horizon. Let us send this usury out as well. The star of the sea is far out on the horizon. Let us send this evil spirit out as well.

29 *Carregador* removes the *ebó*:

He is going to take away the smell, Exú *ke-re-ke-re**.

30 O Santo Antonio tie the fellow up, O on his way. O Santo Antonio tie the fellow up, O don't let him come.

31 Fumigation:

Our Lady incensed her Blessed Son to smell sweet, but I incense these children that the evil may go out and happiness enter.

32 Evil, leave these bodies. These bodies belong to the Virgin Mary. As the Virgin Mary incenses her blessed Son that he may smell sweet, so I incense my children to drive all evil far away, and to attract good all about them. In the name of Almighty God, the current of the stars and of the waters. I went into Noah's ark and locked you in with the key of the sanctuary.

I.2 and C.6 both considered the 'complex' *ebó* (*trabalho*, *limpeza de corpo*) to be the most powerful and effective way of combating undesirable forces that may make a person ill. C.2, however, looked upon the 'complex' *ebó* as being one of a series of rituals that, if conducted in unison, constituted an infallible method of treatment. The *ebó* should, in his opinion, be followed by three further rituals if it is to succeed.

The *pai de santo* should hold a *sessão espírita* (spirit session), preferably on the same day as the *trabalho*, as a preliminary to the ritual known as *limpeza dos astros* (cleansing by the stars). As many mediums as possible associated with the cult house attend and sit together round a table. The colour of their clothes should normally be white, but sometimes, particularly if the *sessão* coincides with a feast day, some of the mediums may wear a shirt and/or a dress of the colour usually associated with their *orixá*. It is customary for the *pai* to issue each medium with a short white overall tied at the back as well as a belt and a white linen cap, and these may be discarded during possession in favour of clothing more suited to the *orixá* in question. There are usually one or two candles alight on the table, various vases of flowers (usually chinchirinchee and/or white roses) and in front of the *pai* a *copo de vidência*. This is a glass containing different coloured stones and an aluminium cross, and filled with clear water. The *pai* uses it periodically during the *sessão* for divination, and may use the water inside it for washing the faces of those present, particularly those that are to be cured.

The mediums and patients sit round the table in such a way that each patient has a medium on either side. The *presidente* exhorts everybody to be silent and to concentrate on attracting good spirits, known as *irmãos de luz* (brothers of light) or *espíritos*, to the table. Although the spirits are referred to by both these terms, however, they invariably turn out to be familiar *orixás* or *caboclo* spirits, and I never witnessed a medium being possessed by an unfamiliar spirit when the primary purpose of the *sessão* was that of curing.[34] When all the mediums are possessed, the *pai* (also possessed) instructs everyone at the table to hold hands so that the *corrente* (current) or power emanating from each spirit may pass through the bodies of the patients. As already mentioned (page 103 n. 41), this action is described by the verb *encorrentar* (to pass a current).

As the different spirits take possession of their mediums the following dialogue takes place between the spirit speaking through the medium, and the onlookers:

SPIRIT: Praised be Our Lord Jesus Christ.
ONLOOKERS: Let him be praised for ever.
SPIRIT: Praised be Our Lord Jesus Christ.
ONLOOKERS: Let him be praised for ever.
SPIRIT: May the peace of Our Lord Jesus Christ pour over all your heads.
ONLOOKERS: So be it.

Directly after this dialogue, the spirit is greeted with one or more incantations that belong specially to him.

When all the spirits have been honoured in this way (and this may take two or three hours), the *pai* hands each person present a lighted candle and leads the way outside. Seven candles are symbolically wiped over the patient's body and then lit at the entrance to the property.[35]

The *pai*, holding a crucifix over the patient's head, says the following prayer:

God salute you stars. God salute you waters. God salute you virgin jungle. From the stars comes a message, and from the waters comes a power, the waters of the sacred sea to defend you, opening your ways in the name of Oxalá, Oxossi, Ogun, Yemanjá and Abaluayé.

This is followed by the following spontaneous prayer:

These lights[36] are going to light her paths. My brothers, I ask all of you in the name of the phalanx of the divine Holy Spirit, to lift your lights that the sufferings of this creature may also be raised aloft, that Jesus may bless her, since she has come in search of His mercy. Father sublime, beloved master, pour your beneficent essence over the head of this creature and all of you present. Oh Father, I beg you from the depths of my heart, Oxossi Mineiro[37] at this holy table, cast a compassionate eye on these sons of yours present here, paying homage to the stars that they may bless this child and all who are here.

All those present now place their candles on the ground to form a close circle round the patient. The *pai* then makes the patient repeat the following three times:

I am saved, I shall be saved.

Each time the words are said, the patient must jump in the air. The patient then repeats after the *pai*:

With the force of Oxalá, the divine master, Ogun, Oxossi with all his phalanx and Abaluayé.

and immediately afterwards jumps out of the circle. Everyone present claps.

The *limpeza dos astros* just described is now followed by a *limpeza das águas* (cleansing by the waters). The timing of the ceremony is important, because it should coincide exactly with the full moon and when the tide is beginning to turn from flood to ebb. This means that the whole series of rituals, beginning with the 'complex' *ebó*, should be arranged in such a manner that they coincide as closely as possible with the full moon. In the series of rituals witnessed, the 'complex' *ebó* was performed on the day when a full moon was expected at night and the timing of the *limpeza dos astros* was fixed so that it would be over well before the tide turned.

All the mediums (many of whom are still in trances), the patients and the onlookers process down to the beach with a series of dishes of food prepared specially for the goddesses of water (Yemanjá and Oxun).[38] This offering is known as the patient's *obrigação* (obligation), and it may include animals sacred to Yemanjá and Oxun if the patient's finances permit, though it more often takes the form of separate plates of black beans, brown beans, maize flour, cooked rice and at least three *acaçá*. These ingredients are wiped over the patient's body in the order given, in accordance with the established progression from dark to lighter colours and from raw to cooked food. Each plate is then placed on the surface of the water and allowed to sink, but sometimes, if the patient is restricted financially, the plate need not be offered as well as the food. This ritual is not accompanied by incantations or prayers, but, later on, in the cult house a *festa* (feast, celebration) is held to celebrate the successful completion of the rituals.

The following morning an offering is made by the patient to the *caboclo* spirits of the jungle, thereby requesting them to join with all the other forces already invoked and to contribute towards bringing about a cure. The *pai* cooks a pumpkin (provided by the patient), and then hollows it out and fills it with honey and flowers. The patient next speaks into it and makes his or her special request to the *caboclos*. The two halves are then joined together and left by the patient in the jungle in a circle made by twenty-one candles.

CONCLUSION

This study of *curandeirismo* has required the inclusion of an appraisal of *Candomblé de caboclo* since so many of the curing practices discussed find their origins in one or more of the different religious currents that have contributed towards *Candomblé de caboclo*. The African influence stands out as being the strongest—predictably so, in that from early days there were numerically considerably more African peoples in the area than members of any other group, and today it is noticeable that people are mainly of African stock. The African tradition of worship through the medium assuming the identity of his or her *orixá* (i.e. falling into a trance) is still extremely common, and, as has been seen, it is at the basis of many of the thaumaturgic healing methods described in this study in that the patient often consults not only the *curandeiro* but also the *curandeiro*'s *orixá* for advice about a cure. This is particularly the case in a *trabalho*, which is always preceded by a *consulta*, during which instructions for the *trabalho* are given (see Chapter XI).

This comparative ease in falling into a trance has kept very much alive the notion that man is protected by his *orixá*, who, if displeased in any way, could send illness or any form of indisposition as a result of his displeasure. The *orixás* must therefore be treated in the correct ritual fashion or all manner of misfortunes may follow. Ritual observance of taboo is most strictly followed, this being the case also among adherents to the *Candomblé de caboclo* cult, even though their taboos are less severe than in more traditional houses.

The European contribution (pre-Christian, Christian and Spiritist) is also substantial, and this is the result of a variety of factors. From the beginning of colonization, it was considered a mark of social superiority among the slaves to be baptized into the Catholic religion, and, as miscegenation took place, to adopt more and more Portuguese customs. Catholicism has always been the official religion of Brazil, while African religions have periodically been persecuted, so all aspects of Catholicism have been allowed uninterrupted propagation. Moreover, whereas immigration from Africa stopped with the abolition of slavery, immigration from Catholic European countries (mainly Portugal, Spain and Italy) has been continuous right up to the present day. This has allowed a constant renewal process of popular Catholic and folkloric elements, since many of the practices of European origin as described in this study are still found in certain parts of Spain, particularly Galicia, and Portugal, especially the northern province of Entre Douro e Minho that borders with Galicia, as is shown by fieldwork observation and documentary evidence in the text.

Spiritism has provided a further form of renewal in that it is in many ways an evolved type of *Candomblé*, involving, as it does, the possession of mediums by spirits. In addition, Spiritism, with its central preoccupation with healing, has in this locality introduced into *curandeirismo* the concept of healing by way of 'group therapy'. The idea behind *encorrentar* (see page 103 n. 41), which requires the patient to join hands with all possessed mediums present, is that the *corrente* (current) from the spirits should flow right through the patient and cleanse him of any evil influence that may be making him ill.

The spirits, known as *irmãos de luz*, are rarely anything but traditional *orixás* and/or *caboclo* spirits, but the mediums are precluded from dancing when possessed until all the normal curing procedures have taken place. The more sedate atmosphere of the spirit session, involving, as it does, the mediums sitting at a table and concentrating on curing, has given a totally new dimension to the faithful's relationship with the *orixás*. Instead of the *orixá* being in complete control of the situation, with all present doing his will (during a *Candomblé* celebration, for example), he is, in the spirit session, firmly manipulated by the *presidente*, whose job it is to ensure that all the curing procedures are completed within a certain fixed time limit. Spirit sessions are always held at regular intervals: C.2's was held every Thursday at 8 p.m., while I.6's took place only on the first Monday and last Thursday of the month at 5 p.m. and was allowed to proceed for no longer than one hour on each occasion. This enforced formality of the spirit session, with its strict timetable and lack of drums and dancing as a means of summoning the *orixás*, constitutes the main difference between it and a *festa* (feast), which involves a great deal more physical activity and has no time limitations imposed upon it. The spirit session requires the *orixás*, on the guidance of the *presidente*, to concentrate all their energies on one specific purpose at regular intervals and for a carefully controlled period of time.

The indigenous contribution to curing ritual, when compared with the African and European contributions just mentioned, is relatively small. This is curious, in that *caboclo* spirits appear to be becoming more and more popular among cult members, and so, at first sight, the indigenous element appears to be larger than in fact it is. But this popularity of the *caboclo* is based mainly on such factors as compatibility and economics rather than an inclination on the part of cult members towards indigenous cultures in preference to others. The *caboclo* is more approachable and less detached than his African counterpart, who is generally much more aloof and considerably more demanding. While the African *orixá* requires his followers to own a lavish costume and make extravagant sacrifices at specific times during the year, the *caboclo* is less exigent and renders it much easier, especially in economic terms, for his devotees to fulfil their obligations.

Another reason for the popularity of the *caboclos* is the comparatively recent resurgence of Tupi culture among intellectuals in an attempt to establish a national identity. This movement gained a hold in the 1920s, and brought a revival in indigenous art forms, history and language to such an extent that, for some years, a serious attempt was made to establish Tupi Guarani as the language of Brazilian intellectuals. The reappraisal of Tupi culture permeated through to other strata of society, and whatever indigenous element there is present in *Candomblé de caboclo* stems primarily from this and is not a survival of a contribution made by the Indian at the beginning of colonization. The Indian's role on the plantations was very soon taken over completely by the African slave, the result being that the Indian drifted definitively away from population centres and back into the interior.

There is still little documentary evidence concerning Indian cultures in Brazil of the type which could provide an adequate insight into their religions and curing practices, and this makes it all the more difficult satisfactorily to evaluate what indigenous contributions there may have been to *curandeirismo* and associated rituals as discussed in this study. There are, admittedly, some elements which may stem from an indigenous source. These were mentioned above at the time of discussion, and are principally *sacudida*, fumigation (mainly with tobacco smoke) and ritual baths (presumably of the pure-water variety, since there appears to be no specific reference to any form of indigenous herbal bath). Conversely, these practices were equally common to European and African cultures, and, as our evaluation has shown, they show a marked tendency to have developed without much reliance on any significant indigenous contribution. The European ritual *reza*, involving the brushing of leaves over the patient's body to the accompaniment of a prayer, is closely akin to the *sacudida* (and probably derives from it), but the prayers accompanying such rituals are mainly European (No. 37 (page 103) being the only exception in which there is mention of a *caboclo* spirit). Similarly, the prayers for the *sacudida* transcribed in Chapter V show mainly a pre-occupation with African and Catholic elements. Moreover, the herbs used in these rituals are so employed either because of their affinity with specific African *orixás* or on account of their traditional use in Europe for such purposes. The indigenous contribution to herb lore is minimal and restricted, in the main, to the provision of Tupi names to some plants.

There are, however, a number of reasons why European and African elements should have syncretized and developed as markedly as they clearly have done. First, as mentioned above (page 5ff.), many of the Africans who came from Portuguese colonies were already familiar with Portuguese culture and the language, and were as a result able to settle down more easily after their transition to the new colony of Brazil. In addition to this, the African was able to discern considerable similarities between his religion and Catholicism. Not only could he reconcile the *orixás* with the Catholic saints, but he could also identify with many characteristic Catholic tenets (for example, the guardian angel; the mother cult; the intercessor/confessor figure; fumigation; certain taboos such as fasting and abstinence). Moreover, the Catholic idea of the devil and his connection with hell-fire appeared to be an extension of the African Exú, who was believed to have originally brought fire, though in this case for the benefit of mankind. The basic dualism in Exú could very easily be extended into a Catholic context by linking the demoniacal side of his character to the devil, and the more beneficent side to Saint Michael the Archangel, who drove the fallen angel to hell. This additional link with Saint Michael is found mainly in the south of Brazil (particularly in Rio de Janeiro and São Paulo), though Exú commands considerable respect in Bahia, as exemplified by the terms used to refer to him: *o chefe* (the chief) and *o chefão* (the big chief). Exú's ambivalent personality is a succinct embodiment of the forces of both good and evil, and he is both the agent that may be invoked to put evil on a victim and the agent that is invoked to remove it.

In addition to these religious similarities, there were also basic cultural similarities between Europe and Africa. The linking of herbs to gods in ancient Egypt is virtually identical to the Yoruba tradition, whereby specific herbs are placed under the control of specific *orixás*. The astrologers' idea that a planet may bring disease if in a certain position in the heavens, and that the herbs linked to it can also bring healing, flourished in Europe at the time of colonization. These notions coincided with the Yoruba idea that each *orixá* controls a certain part of the body and can therefore bring either harm or healing to it depending on the way the *orixá* in question is treated. Similarly, African taboos with regard to the collection of herbs were closely akin to the astrologers' insistence on harmony among the spheres before certain herbs could be picked for specific purposes.

The influence of Islam was also common in many different ways to both Europe and Africa. Amulets such as the pentangle and the *breve* were brought over simultaneously by both the Portuguese and certain of the Africans, showing a common origin in the Moslem concern with the power of cabbalistic signs and of the written word.

These basic and deep-rooted similarities between the two main cultures that constitute *Candomblé de caboclo* may be behind certain common characteristics which exist in the different curing methods described in this study. All the methods (namely, *sacudida*, fumigation, ritual baths, the use of *pemba* and amulets, the curing prayer, and the *ebó*) involve ridding the patient of the force of evil that is the cause of the indisposition, so that the body may be left ritually clean and able to heal itself. But one of the fundamental characteristics of many of the rituals is that, after the evil has been expelled, a similar ritual with modifications (especially of ingredients employed) is enacted to attract forces of good. Hence, in fumigation, ingredients to expel evil are employed first while the person fumigating moves through the house from the back door to the front. Then the ingredients are changed for those which attract only good forces, and fumigation continues from the front door to the back, thereby bringing all the good forces into the house. This process of attracting good by the use of specific substances subsequent to the expulsion of evil is also followed in the case of ritual baths.

The main substances employed are herbs, and the reason for using a particular herb is based on the character and the function in myth of the *orixá* who controls it. The use of herbs can be fairly complex, as in the case of the numerous combinations for ritual baths, or quite simple, as in the case of the *reza*, in which usually only one herb is employed during the ritual. In all cases, however, the evil is first expelled. C.5 particularly emphasized the importance of first ridding the body of evil before attracting forces of good, his main point being that good forces have the characteristic of 'sealing' the body for a while against evil forces. Hence, if an evil force is not first of all got rid of, it will remain inside and the patient's indisposition will steadily worsen.

Fumigation and the ritual bath both have this characteristic of being able to expel and attract forces (*afastar/atrair*; *descarga/desenvolvimento*). Other methods of cure follow the same basic pattern of first expelling evil and then, towards the end of the ritual, attracting good, usually by means of fumigation, a ritual bath and/or application of *pemba*. This is the case in *sacudida*, which must be followed by fumigation (first to *afastar* and then to *atrair*); but it is seen most clearly in the 'complex' *ebó*, which involves a whole series of different actions designed primarily to remove the evil and destroy it (for example, cutting with scissors certain of the ingredients, sacrificing the scapegoat), and these are followed by fumigation, ritual baths and the application of *pemba*. In the case of amulets, the evil is first attracted to the amulet before entering the body, and is then rendered harmless by the amulet's shape or smell, or the substance of which it is composed.

All the methods of cure discussed involve the spoken or sung recitation of a prayer or incantation at some stage during the ritual. *Pemba* and amulets also are manufactured to the accompaniment of a prayer or incantation. *Patuás/breves* always contain a written prayer or charm together with their other ingredients.

Many of the prayers and incantations transcribed in the text show a marked reliance on the European tradition, though a number of the incantations that accompany the 'complex' *ebós* witnessed are in the original African language. The African content of such incantations is likely to diminish steadily in future as the *caboclo* element becomes more pronounced and as the movement away from traditional *Candomblé* continues. Younger *mães* and *pais de santo* who have been brought up fully in the *caboclo* tradition (for instance, C.9 and C.11) conduct most ceremonies in the vernacular and never converse in an African language. Some of those who have retained a certain amount of the African language in their incantations are unable to give a translation into Portuguese. (See, for example, some of the prayers/incantations transcribed in Chapter XI.)

The movement away from traditional *Candomblé* implies a movement away from Africa and towards Europe, represented chiefly by Spiritism. African religions in Brazil were, from early colonial days, viewed as unacceptable and undesirable (and often incomprehensible) since they stemmed only from the slave population, which lay at the very bottom of the social scale. On account of this social stigma, many Africans, as already pointed out, sought a Catholic baptism so as to cease being considered pagan and accordingly socially inferior. This view of African religion prevailed after Abolition, and was the underlying factor behind much of the official persecution in the first half of the twentieth century. More recently, however, following the advent of Spiritism, with its clear European origins and its incorporation into traditional *Candomblé* in the genesis of *Candomblé de caboclo*, basically African cults have become more socially acceptable and have for many lost the social stigma originally associated with them.

Spiritist-influenced *Candomblé de caboclo* permits the traditional worship of the *orixás* in a considerably more dignified way, with mediums often working seated at a table rather than dancing. For others, however, the social stigma still survives: the three patients mentioned in Chapter XI (C.2) refused to allow their faces to be photographed because they were afraid of the photographs being published. These patients belonged to the professional class by training: a doctor, a teacher and a lawyer, and for such people it is unlikely that *curandeirismo* of this nature will ever lose its stigma, since it is perpetuated principally by the lower socio-economic classes, and *curandeiros* tend to come from poor backgrounds. However, what unites these classes is a faith in thaumaturgic curing which permeates society at all levels and spans a variety of religious beliefs from the orthodox and long-established Roman Catholic acceptance of miraculous cures to the internationally renowned 'operations' of faith healers like José Arigó. In Bahia in 1973–4, people both inside and outside *Candomblé* circles, including professional people, spoke of the feats performed by *o médico invisível*, a certain Doctor Fritz, a doctor of German origin who continued to operate after his death by giving precise instructions to mediums through whom he worked, directing complex operations step by step.[1]

Other quasi-religious and messianic movements have also sprung up in the wake of Spiritism, placing a similar emphasis on curing among their activities, and these have attracted, on the one hand, those unable to afford medical aid in the first place, and, on the other, those for whom conventional medicine can afford no further relief. In the latter case, *curandeirismo* and group therapy based on religious worship are seen as a last resort, while in other cases they may complement conventional medical treatment. I.2 often advised patients to consult a doctor for conditions she clearly recognized to be beyond her powers of alleviation, but recommended a ritual *trabalho* so as to 'desenvolver' the doctor's spirit that he might be enlightened sufficiently to make an accurate diagnosis and prescribe a satisfactory cure. This having been successfully accomplished, the patient might feel obliged to complement the medical treatment with another *trabalho* or a ritual sacrifice of thanksgiving to assure the permanence of the cure. Professional medicine and folk medicine are therefore not always easily distinguishable, and a cure may be attributed to the complementary action of both. By allying itself with professional medicine in this way, *curandeirismo* assures its self-perpetuation. Just as votive offerings to Catholic saints have preceded and followed medical intervention, so the same process takes place with the *orixás*, and medical skill can be attributed to the guiding hand of the *orixás* whose power remains undiminished in the face of modern scientific knowledge.

Coexistence and interaction therefore appear to be the means of safeguarding and guaranteeing the continuation both of African-based religion and popular medicine in the Recôncavo: African deities continue to be revered publicly in the guise of Catholic saints, and propitiation of the *orixás* by the faithful assures their favourable influence in effecting a cure, when invoked by the *curandeiro*, either directly or via the vehicle of the professional doctor.

APPENDIX ONE

THE BRAZILIAN PORTUGUESE NAMES OF HERBS, PLANTS AND TREES

The herbs, plants and trees are listed alphabetically according to the following scheme:

1. Botanical name(s)
2. *Orixá*(s) by whom controlled
3. *Sacudida*
4. Fumigation: *afastar*; *atrair*. These will be abbreviated to *af.*; *at.*
5. Ritual baths: *desenvolvimento*; *descarga*; *abó*; *amasi*. These will be abbreviated to *desen.*; *desc.*; *ab.*; *am.*
6. *Pemba*
7. *Reza*
8. Taboos
9. Other observations

In cases where information was unobtainable, the relevant number has been omitted. When there is apparent disparity of views, reference is made to the relevant informants.

Wherever possible, suggestions have been made as to the botanical identity of the plants, but it must be emphasized that this information has been gleaned mainly from botanical dictionaries and other published sources and should be used only as a guide to probable true identity. Popular names for herbs vary considerably throughout Brazil, and sources hence often give two or more botanical names. All possible alternatives have been given wherever this has been deemed necessary. For ease of reference, Appendix Two lists these botanical names alphabetically with their probable Brazilian Portuguese equivalents.

Abre caminhos
1. *Kanimia* Gardn.
2. Ogun
3. Yes
4. *Af.*
5. *Desen.; desc.*
6. No
7. No
8. Pick before sunrise
9. The name *abre caminhos* is given

to this herb because Ogun 'opens the ways' (i.e. resolves difficulties) with his sword. Can be included in *patuás*

Acoco

2. All the *orixás*
3. No
4. *Af.*; *at.* (C.5); no (C.1)
5. *Desen.*; *desc.*; *ab.*; *am.*
6. Yes
7. No
8. Best to pick on first Friday of Lent (C.5); pick only on Thursday or Friday (C.1)
9. For planting ritual, see page 28. It will die if touched by someone who is ritually unclean

Agua de Levante

1. *Amomum cardamomum* L.; *Renealmia brasiliensis* Schum.
2. Yansan (1.2): Oxun, Yemanjá (S.6); Ogun (C.1)
3. Yes (C.5); no (C.1)
4. *At.* (C.5); no (C.1)
5. *Desen.*; *desc.*; *am.*
6. Yes
7. Yes
8. On picking, leave an offering of money near the plant. This herb is called *erva paga* ('paid-for herb')

Alecrim

1. *Rosmarinus officinalis* L.
2. Yemanjá
3. No
4. *At.*
5. *Desen.*; *ab.*
6. Yes
7. Yes
8. None
9. A cross of *alecrim* may be sewn on the outside of a *patuá*

Alfavaca

1. *Ocimum fluminensis* V.
2. Ibeji
3. No
4. No
5. *Desen.*; *desc.*

Alfazema

1. *Lavandula spica* L.; *Lavandula vera*
2. Oxun, Yemanjá (I.1, S.6); Yansan (C.1)
4. *Af.*; *at.*
5. *Desen.*; *desc.*
6. Yes
7. Yes, but rarely (I.2); no (C.1)
8. Pick before sunset, or before midday to attract good, after sunset to get rid of evil forces
9. It is used particularly to fumigate a newly born baby and all the clothing worn by both the baby and the mother during the first seven days after birth. (See also Lima 1946:86–7; Câmara Cascudo 1951:84)

Aluman

1. *Veronia bahiensis* Toledo
2. Omolú, Yansan
3. Yes
5. *Desen.*; *desc.*; *ab.*
8. Pick on Monday
9. Used to cure mental disturbance, three leaves being placed underneath the patient's pillow

Angélica

1. *Guettarda angelica* Mart.
2. Oxun
3. No
4. No
5. *Desen.*; *desc.*; *ab.*
6. Yes
7. No
8. Leave money next to plant when picking
9. Also called *angélica do sertão*

Apetite

1. *Allium oleraceum* L; *Allium schoenoprasum* L.

9. Leaves passed by themselves over the body will help to get rid of an *egun* (C.6)

Araçá de porco

1. *Psidium araçá* Rad; *Psidium cuneatum* Camb.; *Psidium humile* Vel.
5. *Desen.*
8. Picker must not have consumed alcohol within previous twenty-four hours

Arco de barris

1. *Sparattanthelium botucudorum*
2. Omolú
3. No
5. *Desen.* (I.2); no (C.1)
7. No

Aroeira

1. *Schinus molle* L.
2. Exú (I.2); Omolú, Yansan (C.1); Oxossi (C.6)
3. Yes
4. No
5. *Desen.; desc.; ab.; am.*
7. No
8. Pick at 5 a.m.

Arruda

1. *Ruta graveolens* L.
2. Omolú, Yansan (C.1)
3. No (I.2); yes (C.1)
4. *Af.; at.*
5. *Desen.; desc.; ab.*
7. Yes
8. Pick when temperature is cool (i.e. early in the morning)
9. This herb is dealt with at length on page 24. Used for the manufacture of *figas* (see page 74). Three leaves may be worn behind the ear as an amulet (see page 80)

Assapeixe branco

1. *Vernonia membranacia* Gardn.
2. Yansan

Avenca

1. *Adiantum capillus-veneris* L.
2. Oxun, Yemanjá (I.2, S.6); Naná (C.1)
9. This plant will wilt if looked at by a victim of the evil eye. It must be looked after by only one person

Açafrão

1. *Crocus sativus* L.
4. *At.*

Banana

1. Various species of the *Musa* genus
3. Yes

Barba de bode

1. *Cyperus compressus* L.
3. Yes
5. *Desc.*
6. Yes

Barba de São Pedro

1. *Polygala paniculata* L.
2. Omolú
5. *Desen.*
7. Yes
8. Pick only half a leaf at a time

Barquinho de Noé

1. *Rhoeo discolor* Hanc.
2. Oxalá
5. *Desen.*
8. Pick very early in the morning

Bejerecum

1. Possibly *Xylopia*
4. *Af.*
5. *Desc.*
6. Yes
9. If the seed is collected between Maundy Thursday and Good Friday, it can be used in a *patuá* or worn round the neck as an amulet (see page 80)

Betis cheiroso

1. *Piper eucaliptifolium* Rudge.
2. Naná (I.2); Oxun, Yemanjá (S.6); Ogun, Yansan (C.1)
3. Yes
5. *Desen.; desc.; ab.; am.*

7. Yes
8. Pick between 3 and 4 a.m.
9. Also known as *betis branco*

Bonina
1. *Mirabilis jalapa* L.
2. Oxun
5. *Desen.; am.*
8. Pick early, between 3 and 4 a.m.

Brilhantina
1. *Pilea microphylla*
2. Oxun, Yemanjá
5. *Desen.; desc.*
8. Pick early, between 3 and 4 a.m.

Caiçara
1. *Solanum pulverulentum*
2. Omolú
3. Yes
5. *Desc.*
7. Yes

Cajá
1. *Spondias cytherea*
5. *Ab.; am.*
9. *Abó* mixture suspended on the trunk

Canela de velho
1. *Zinnia elegans* Jacq.; *Miconia albicans*
2. Omolú
5. *Desen.; desc.*
8. Pick on Monday
9. Leaf placed on top of head to cure madness

Cansanção
1. *Jatropha urens* L; *Jatropha oligandra* Muell.
2. Exú
5. *Desc.*
6. Yes, but only *pemba de Exú*
9. *Cansanção* stings, and disobedient initiates are obliged, while in a trance, to roll on a bed of *cansanção* by way of punishment. When picked with the left hand, it can only be used for evil ends

Capianga
1. *Vismia brasiliensis* Chois.
2. Yansan (I.2); Ogun (S.6)
3. Yes
5. *Desc.; ab.*
6. Yes
7. Yes
8. Pick on Wednesdays

Capiçoba
1. *Polygonum acre* H.B.K.
2. Ogun
5. *Desen.*

Capim de caboclo
1. *Andropogon saccharoides* Sw.; *Andropogon sorghum* Brot.; *Andropogon nardus* L.
2. Yansan (C.2)
4. *At.*
5. *Desen.; desc.*
8. Pick between 5 and 9.30 a.m.

Capim estrela
1. *Dichromena ciliata* Vahl.
2. Ibeji
5. *Desc.*
8. Pick on a Monday

Capim santo
1. *Kyllinga odorata* Vahl.
2. Ibeji
5. *Ab.*, but rarely
8. Pick on a Friday

Carqueja
1. *Baccharis genistifolia* D.C.
5. *Desen.*
8. Pick on a Friday

Catinga de crioula
1. *Stachys fluminensis*
2. Oxun
5. *Desen.; ab.*
8. Pick on Tuesdays as early as possible
9. Also called *quese-quese*

Catinga de porco
1. *Caesalpinia pyramidalis* Tul.

2. Yansan (S.6); Omolú (C.6)
4. *At.*
5. *Desen.; ab.*
9. Also known as *catingueira*. May also be included in a *patuá*

Coerana

1. *Cestrum laevigatum* Sch.
2. Omolú (I.2, S.6); Ogun, Yansan, Omolú and Exú (C.1)
3. Yes
5. *Desc.; ab.*
7. Yes
9. Used particularly for driving away an *egun*. May not be used in *sacudida* where patient belongs to Yansan (see page 33). If picked between 9 a.m. and midnight, it belongs to Exú and can be used only for evil; if picked between 4 and 9 a.m., it can only be used for good purposes

Cordão de São Francisco

1. *Leonurus sibiricus* L.
2. Ogun
3. Yes
5. *Desen.*
7. Yes
9. Also called *cordão de frade*

Corredeira

1. *Euphorbia pillulifera* L.
2. Exú
4. *Af.*
5. *Desc.*
6. Yes, but only *pemba de Exú*
8. Pick only at full moon
9. Leaf placed under trays of merchandise by street vendors to promote sales

Dandá

1. *Cyperus rotundus* L.; *Cyperus longus* L.; *Cyperus esculentus* L.
4. *At.* but rarely
6. Yes
8. Pick in Holy Week, if possible on Good Friday
9. Used in *patuás* and may be sewn into a baby's clothing to protect against evil. A small piece is often placed in the mouth to protect against evil when it is supposed that evil influence is at its strongest (e.g. during a curing ritual)

Dendê

1. *Elaeis guineensis* Jacq.
9. Widely used in *Candomblé* ritual and constitutes an important part of the *pade de Exú* (see page 32, n. 5). *Abó* mixture suspended on the trunk

Erva cidreira

1. *Melissa officinalis* L.
5. *Desen.*

Erva de passarinho

1. *Struthanthus vulgaris; Struthanthus brasiliensis*
2. Xangô (S.6); Exú (C.1)
5. *Desen.* (S.6); no (C.1)
6. Yes, but *pemba de Exú* only (C.1)

Eva Santa Maria, see *Mastruz*

Espada de Ogun

1. *Sansevieria zeylanica* Willd.
2. Ogun
3. Yes
4. No
5. *Desc.; ab.*
8. Pick before 6 a.m. or directly after 6 p.m. (i.e. just before sunset).

Espada de Oxossi

1. *Sansevieria trifasciata laurentii*
2. Oxossi
3. Yes
5. *Ab.*

Espada de Yansan

2. Yansan
3. Yes
5. *Ab.*

Espinho cheiroso

1. *Xanthoxylum rhoifolium* Lam.
2. Naná

4. *Af.*
5. *Desen.; desc.; ab.*
6. Yes
8. Pick on Saturdays

Favaquinha de cobra
1. *Monnieria trifolia* L.
2. Yemanjá (S.6); Naná (C.1)
4. *At.*
5. *Desen.*
8. Pick between 4 and 6.30 a.m.
9. Also called *folha de vidro*

Favico
9. A seed that is worn round the neck as an amulet (see page 80)

Fedegoso
1. *Cassia occidentalis* L.
4. *Af.*
5. *Desc.*

Folha da Costa
1. *Kalanchoe brasiliensis*
2. Oxun
5. *Desen.; ab.; am.*
7. Yes, but rarely
9. Also known as *folha de bori*, and used during this ceremony. It is also used during most ceremonies involving sacrifice (C.6) (see page 123)

Folha de algodão
1. *Gossypium hirsutum* L.
2. Oxalá (Bastide 1961:163)
4. *Af.*
5. *Desc.*

Folha de laranja da terra
1. *Citrus aurantium* L.
2. Yemanjá
4. *Af.; at.* (not the leaf, but the skin of the fruit)
5. *Desen.*

Folha de limão
1. *Citrus medica* L.
2. Exú
4. *At.*
5. *Desen.*
6. Yes, but only for *pemba de Exú*

Folha de mamona
1. *Ricinus communis* L.
2. Yansan
4. *At.*
5. *Desen.*

Folha de Marcela
1. *Achyrocline satureioides* D.C.
5. *Desen.*
9. Also called *Marcela do campo*, *Marcela galega* and *Marcela de colchão*

Folha de neve
1. *Hyptis pectinata* Poit.
2. Naná (S.6).; Yemanjá (C.1)
4. *At.*
5. *Desen.; desc.*
6. Yes
7. Yes, but rarely
8. Pick between 4 and 6 a.m., and certainly no later than 6 a.m.

Folha santa
1. *Peltodon radicans*
2. Omolú
4. *Af.*
5. *Desc.*
9. Also known as *rabulho de cachorro*

Folha de urubú
1. *Pothos quadrangularis; Coccoloba sagitifolia; Coccoloba latifolia*
2. Ibeji
3. Yes
4. No
5. *Desc.*
6. Yes, but only *pemba de Exú* (C.1)
7. No

Fruta da ciência
9. It can be worn round the neck as an amulet (see page 80). Also known as *tontiça*

Fruta de São Cipriano
8. It should not be picked up but

allowed to fall naturally from the tree.
9. It may be used as an amulet to protect against the evil eye if it falls with the concave side facing upwards and if it is picked up by a man. If the convex side faces upwards, it may be used for evil, but only if picked up by a woman (see pages 26 and 80)

Fumo brabo
1. *Elephantopus scaber* L.
4. No.
5. *Desc.*

Gameleira
1. *Ficus doliaria* M.
2. Exú; Omolú
3. Yes
4. *Af.; At.*
5. *Desc.*
6. Yes, but only *pemba de Exú*
7. Yes, but rarely

Girassol
1. *Helianthus annuus* L.
2. Oxalá
4. *At.*
5. *Desen.*

Guiné
1. *Petiveria alliacea* L.
2. Omolú
3. Yes
4. *Af.* (S.6)
5. *Desc.; ab.*
6. Yes (I.2)
7. Yes
8. Pick on Wednesday, Thursday and Friday (C.1)
9. Generally considered to be one of the principal leaves in the ritual *reza*. Also known as *tipí* and *pipi* (see page 23). Used for the manufacture of *figas* (see page 74). Three leaves may be worn behind the ear as an amulet (see page 80) Can also be included in *patuás*

Hortelã grosso
1. *Mentha viridis* L.
5. *Desen.; desc.*

Imbé
1. *Philodendron imbé* Schott.
9. Used in most rituals to cure victims of the evil eye and *moléstia do ar*

Jaqueira
1. *Artocarpus heterophyllus*
9. *Abó* mixture suspended on the trunk

Jarrinha
1. *Aristolochia cymbifera* Mart.
4. *At.*
5. *Desen.*
8. Pick only Monday, Tuesday and Friday

Jasmin do Plário
1. *Plumeria lutea* R. & P.; *Plumeria aurantia* Lodd.
6. Yes, but only for *pemba de Exú*
9. A lizard (unknown species) that lays eggs in the bark can be grated and used as *pemba de Exú* (see page 69). Also known as *jasmin do Cairo*

Jeribão
1. *Pavonia cancelata*
4. *Af.*
5. *Desc.*

Jitirana
1. Convolvulus contortus Vell.
2. Oxossi
5. *Desen.*

Juiz de paz
1. *Acanthospermum xanthioides* D. C.; *Xanthium spinosum* L.
4. *Af.*
5. *Desc.*

Jurema preta
1. *Mimosa nigra; Acacia hostilis* Benth.; *Acacia jurema* Mart.
2. Omolú

9. Used in *patuás* as general protection against illness (see also Câmara Cascudo 1951: 88–9)

Jerubeba
1. *Solanum paniculatum* L.
3. Yes
4. *Af.*
5. *Desc.*

Lança de Oxalá
2. Oxalá
5. *Desen.; ab.*
9. It should be sown on a Friday in the middle of a pentangle scratched on the ground

Língua de vaca
1. *Talinum patens* Willd.; *Chaptalia tomentosa* Vent.
2. Yemanjá
5. *Desc.*

Lírio branco
1. *Lilium candidum* L.
2. Oxun (I.2); Oxalá (S.6); Yemanjá (C.1)
3. Yes, but rare
4. *Af.*
5. *Desen.; desc.*
7. Yes, but rarely
8. When picking, light a candle at the edge of water

Louco branco
1. *Plumbago scandens* L.
5. *Desen.; desc.*
6. Yes, but *pemba de Exú* only
8. Pick with the left hand and without looking at the bush
9. This is a herb whose properties and use change radically according to the time of day, e.g. it may be employed for good purposes if picked between 5.30 and 5.45 a.m., or 4 and 6.20 p.m.; and for evil purposes if picked between 5.45 and 10 a.m. or from 6.20 p.m. onwards. Cannot be picked for good purposes in November

Macaça
2. Yemanjá; Oxalá
4. *At.*
5. *Desen.; ab.*
7. Yes
9. The plant will wilt if looked at by a victim of the evil eye. It must be looked after by only one person

Malmequer
1. *Wedelia paludosa* D.C.
2. Ogun; Oxun (Bastide 1961: 165)
4. *Af.*
5. *Desen.; desc.*
8. Pick very early in the morning

Malva branca
1. *Anacyclus aureus*
2. Omolú; Yemanjá (Lima 1946: 96)
4. *Af.; at.*
5. *Desc.*

Malva risco
1. *Urena lobata* L.; *Sida micrantha* St. Hil.
2. Yemanjá
4. *Af.; at.*
5. *Desen.; desc.*

Manjericão
1. *Ocimum basilicum* L.
2. Yemanjá; Naná; Oxalá; Oxun
4. *At.*
5. *Desen.; desc.; ab.; am.*
6. Yes
7. Yes
8. Pick between 4 and 5.30 a.m.
9. One of the principal herbs used in the *reza* ritual. There are many different types of *manjericão* with similar properties and which go under the following names: *manjericão de Austrália*, *manjericão graúdo*, *manjericão de Itália*, *manjericão de crioula*, *manjericão miúdo*

Manjerona
1. *Marjorana hortensis*

5. *Am.*

Maracujá
1. *Passiflora alata* Ait.; *Passiflora bahiensis* Klotzsch.
2. Naná
5. *Desen.*
8. Before picking, the picker must take a *banho* (water). The picker must not be harbouring any feelings of anger towards anyone or this might prejudice the patient.

Marianinha
1. *Commelina nudiflora* L.; *Commelina communis* V.; *Commelina deficiens*, Heber.; *Commelina virginica* L.
2. Naná
5. *Desen.; desc.*
9. Also known as *trapoeraba*

Maria preta
1. *Blanchetia heterotricha* D.C.
2. Yansan
5. *Desen.; desc.*
7. Yes, particularly for the evil eye

Maricutia
1. *Rutacea*
5. *Desc.*

Mastruz
1. *Chenopodium ambrosioides* L; *Lepidium bonariense* L.
5. *Desen.*
7. Yes
9. Also known as *erva Santa Maria*

Matapasso
1. *Cassia tora* L.
5. *Desen.; desc.*

Melancia da praia
1. *Solanum balbisii* Dum.; *Solanum agrarium* Sendt.
5. *Desc.*

Mentrasto
1. *Ageratum conyzoides* L.
5. *Desc.*
9. Also known as *mentraço*

Muricí
1. *Byrsonima sericia D.C.*
5. *Ab.*
6. Yes

Murta
1. *Myrtus communis* L.
2. Ogun
5. *Desc.*
7. Yes, particularly for the evil eye
8. Pick at 7 a.m. or between 4.30 and 5 p.m.

Murungu
1. *Erythrina mulungu* M.; *Erythrina corallodendron* L.
2. Omolú
5. *Desc.*
8. Pick at 7 a.m. and between 4.30 and 5 p.m.
9. Also called *mulungu*

Narciso branco
1. *Hedychium coronarium* Koen.
2. Oxun, Yemanjá
3. Yes
4. *Af.; at.*
5. *Desen.; desc.; ab.; am.*
6. Yes
7. Yes, but rarely
8. Pick between 4 and 5 a.m.

Nativo
1. *Panicum crus-ardeae* Willd.; *Panicum elongatum* Poir.
2. Naná
7. Yes

Nicurí de caboclo
1. *Cocos coronata* Mart; *Cocos schizophylla* Mart.
2. Yansan
9. The root of this plant is used in certain *caboclo seitas* for divination. It is cut into segments like the *obi* nut, divination being based on the way these segments fall

when thrown. The root is known as *batata de Nicurí* or *batata de ouricuri*

Noz moscada

1. *Myristica fragrans* Houtt.
2. Omolú
4. *Af.*
5. *Desc.*
6. Yes
8. Pick just before the new moon
9. Often hung round the neck on a thread as a means of avoiding *moléstia do ar*

Obi

1. *Cola acuminata* Schott. & Endl.; *Cola vera* Schum.
5. *Ab.; am.*
9. Used in divination

Palma

1. *Opuntia tuna* Mill.; *Opuntia dillenii* Haw.; *Opuntia burbanki*
2. Yansan
5. *Ab.*
8. Pick between 7 and 9.30 a.m. and 4 and 5 p.m.

Pau pombo

1. *Tapirira guianensis* Aubl.
2. Ogun
3. Yes
4. No (S.6); *at.* (I.2) but rarely
5. *Desc.*
6. Yes (I.2), but rarely
7. Yes (I.2), but rarely
9. Also known as *roxomucumba* and *roxuré*

Pinhão branco

1. *Jatropha curcas* L.
5. *Desc.*
7. Yes, particularly for the evil eye

Pinhão roxo

1. *Jatropha gossypifolia* Muell.
2. Omolú; Ogun
5. *Desc.; ab.*
7. Yes
8. Pick between 4 and 6.30 a.m.
9. One of the principal leaves used in the *reza* ritual to cure evil eye and *moléstia do ar*

Pitanga

1. *Eugenia michelii*
2. Oxun; Yemanjá; Naná; Oxossi
3. Yes
4. *Af.* (S.6 only)
5. *Desc.*
9. *Pitanga* is generally associated with good fortune and is often found as a decoration in the home, particularly at Christmas (cf. Lima 1946:99)

Poejo

1. *Mentha pulegium* L.
2. Oxun; Yemanjá
4. *At.* (I.2 only)
5. *Desen.; desc.*
6. Yes, but rarely
7. Yes (I.2), but rarely

Purga do campo

1. *Viola ipecacuanha* L; *Ionidium ipecacuanha* Vent.; *Hybanthus ipecacuanha* Bail.; *Cephaelis ipecacuanha* A. Rich.
2. Oxossi
5. *Desen.*
8. The picker must have been ritually clean for nine days before picking. Only one leaf may be picked at a time
9. A detailed discussion of this herb is given by Gomes 1809 1st edn. 1972: IX–XLI; Vogel 1970: 41

Quioiô

1. *Ocimum guineensis* Sch.
2. Xangô
5. *Desen.; desc.*
7. Yes (C.1 only), particularly for *moléstia do ar*
8. Pick between 7 and 10. 30 a.m.

Quitoco

1. *Pluchea quitoc* D.C.

2. Yemanjá; Oxun; Yansan
3. Yes (I.2 only)
4. *Af.* (S.6 only)
5. *Desen.; desc.*
6. Yes (I.2 only)
7. Yes
8. Pick very early
9. Can be used for evil purposes if found at a crossroads (C.5 only)

Rompegibão

1. *Bumelia sartorum* Mart.
2. Omolú
5. *Desc.*

Sabugueiro

1. *Sambucus australis* L.; *Sambucus nigra* L.
2. Naná; Omolú
5. *Desc.*
7. Yes (I.2), but rarely (cf. Valle 1963: 604)

Salsa da praia

1. *Ipomoea pes-caprae* Forsk.; *Ipomoea littoralis* Boiss.
2. Yemanjá, Oxun
5. *Desen.; desc.*
8. Pick between 4 and 5 a.m. when the tide is coming in

Sambambaia de caboclo

1. *Lygodium polymorphum* H.B.K.
5. *Desc.*

Sangolovo

1. *Costus spicatus* Sw.
2. Oxalá
3. Yes
5. *Desen.; desc.; ab.; am.*
7. Yes (I.2 only), but rarely
8. Pick between 4 and 5.30 a.m.

São Caetano

1. *Momordica charantia* L.
5. *Desc.*

São Gonçalinho

1. *Casearia sylvestre* Sw.; *Casearia. brasiliensis*; *Casearia lingua* Camb.
2. Oxossi; belongs to all the *orixás* but particularly Omolú (C.1); Ibeji (C.2)
3. Yes
4. *Af.; at.* (I.2 only)
5. *Desen.; desc.; ab.; am.*
6. Yes (I.2 only)
7. Yes
8. Pick the day before it is required
9. Often seen with *pitanga* as a decoration at Christmas time to bring good fortune

Sapatinho de Nossa Senhora

1. *Zebrina pendula* Schnitzl.; *Petrea volubilis* Jacq.
2. Oxun, Yemanjá
5. *Desen.; ab.*
8. Pick early in the morning, and only a quarter-leaf at a time
9. Also called *viuvinha*

Sete chagas

1. *Cuphea balsamona* Cham.
2. Omolú; Oxalá; Ogun
4. *Af.* (I.2 only), but rarely
5. *Desen.; desc.*
7. Yes (I.2), but rarely
8. Pick very early with great calm and patience facing the rising sun

Suspiro branco

1. *Gomphrena globosa* L.
2. Yansan
5. *Desc.*
8. Pick between 4 and 5.30 a.m.

Tapa buraco

1. *Acalypha communis* Muell.; *Piper aduncum* Vell.
2. Exú
3. Yes (C.5 only)
5. *Desc.* (I.2 and S.6 only)
6. Yes, but for *pemba de Exú* only
8. Pick at 6 or 12 in the morning or evening

Tapete de Oxalá

1. *Peltodons* sp.

2. Oxalá
3. Yes (C.5 only)
4. *At.*
5. *Desc.; ab.; am.*
7. Yes (C.5 only), particularly for evil eye
8. Pick between 3 and 5 a.m.
9. Used to wash the head of initiates (C.5 only)

Tira teima
1. *Esenbeckia febrifuga* Juss.
2. Ogun
3. Yes (S.6 only)
4. *Af.*
5. *Desen.; desc.; ab.*
6. Yes (I.2 only)
7. Yes (I.2 only), but rarely
8. Pick between 5 and 6 a.m.

Tomba tudo
2. Ogun (S.6); Exú or Ogun (C.1)
5. *Desc.*
6. Yes; *pemba de Exú* only (C.1)
9. When picked at 6 or 12 in the morning or evening, belongs to Exú and may only be used for evil purposes; when picked at other times, belongs to Ogun (C.1)

Tontiça, see *Fruta da ciência*

Trombeta
1. *Datura* sp.
5. *Desen.*

Umburana
1. *Bursera leptophleos*
2. Omolú
8. Pick during the sunset.
9. Hung round the neck on a thread to protect against *moléstia do ar* (see page 80). It may also be included in a *patuá*. Only the nut is used, not the leaf. Also called *imburana*.

Vassourinha de Nossa Senhora
1. *Scoparia dulcis* L.
2. Yemanjá; Oxun; Naná; Omolú
3. Yes (I.2), but rarely
4. *Af.; at.*
5. *Desen.; ab.; am.*
7. Yes, particularly for the evil eye
9. One of the principal leaves used in the *reza* ritual. After use during the ritual, it is believed to wilt if the patient is indeed a victim of the evil eye. Also called *Vassourinha mofina*

Vassourinha de relógio
1. *Sida nudata* Gand.; *Sida acuta; Sida rhombifolia* Burm.; *Baccharis aphylla* D.C.
3. Yes (I.2), but rarely
5. *Desc.*
7. Yes (I.2), but rarely (cf. Vianna Filho 1946:120)
9. Also called *zunzu* or *zanzo*

Velaminho
1. *Croton campestris* St. Hil.
2. Omolú (Bastide 1961:166, 167 n. 53, 193)
3. Yes (C.5)
4. *Af.*
5. *Desc.*; no (S.6)
9. Placed inside pillow to protect against *moléstia do ar*. Also called *velame*

Vencetudo
1. *Rolandra argenta*
2. Ogun
3. Yes (S.6 only)
4. *Af.*
5. *Desen.; desc.; ab.; am.*
6. Yes
8. Pick between 3.30 and 5 a.m.
9. One of the principal leaves used in fumigation. Can also be included in *patuás*

APPENDIX TWO

BOTANICAL NAMES WITH BRAZILIAN PORTUGUESE EQUIVALENTS

Acacia hostilis Benth.: jurema preta
Acacia jurema Mart.: jurema preta
Acalypha communis Muell.: tapa buraco
Acanthospermum xanthioides D.C.: juiz de paz
Achyrocline satureioides D.C.: folha de marcela
Adiantum capillus-veneris L.: avenca
Ageratum conyzoides L.: mentrasto
Allium oleraceum L.: apetite
Allium schoenoprasum L.: apetite
Amomum cardamomum L.: água de levante
Anacyclus aureus: malva branca
Andropogon nardus L.: capim de caboclo
Andropogon saccharoides Sw.: capim de caboclo
Andropogon sorghum Brot.: capim de caboclo
Aristolochia cymbifera Mart.: jarrinha
Artocarpus heterophyllus: jaqueira
Baccharis aphylla D.C.: vassourinha de relógio
Baccharis genistifolia D.C.: carqueja
Blanchetia heterotricha D.C.: Maria preta
Bumelia sartorum Mart.: rompegibão
Bursera leptophleos: umburana
Byrsonima sericia D.C.: muricí
Caesalpinia pyramidalis Tul.: catinga de porco
Casearia brasiliensis: São Gonçalinho
Casearia lingua Camb.: São Gonçalinho
Casearia sylvestre Sw.: São Gonçalinho
Cassia occidentalis L.: fedegoso
Cassia tora L.: matapasso
Cephaelis ipecacuanha A.Rich.: purga do campo
Cestrum laevigatum Sch.: *coerana*
Chaptalia tomentosa Vent.: língua de vaca
Chenopodium ambrosioides L.: mastruz
Citrus aurantium L.: folha de laranja da terra

Citrus medica L.: folha de limão
Coccoloba latifolia: folha de urubú
Coccoloba saggitifolia: folha de urubú
Cocos coronata Mart.: nicurí de caboclo
Cocos schizophylla Mart.: nicurí de caboclo
Cola acuminata Schott. & Endl.: obi
Cola vera Schum.: obi
Commelina communis V.: marianinha
Commelina deficiens Heber.: marianinha
Commelina nudiflora L. : marianinha
Commelina virginica L.: marianinha
Convolvulus contortus Vell.: jitirana
Costus spicatus Sw.: sangolovo
Crocus sativus L.: açafrão
Croton campestris St Hil.: velaminho
Cuphea balsamona Cham.: sete chagas
Cyperus compressus L.: barba de bode
Cyperus esculentus L.: dandá
Cyperus longus L.: dandá
Cyperus rotundus L.: dandá
Dichromena ciliata Vahl.: capim estrela
Elaeis guineensis Jacq.: dendê
Elephantopus scaber L.: fumo brabo
Erythrina corallodendron L.: murungu
Erythrina mulungu M.: murungu
Esenbeckia febrifuga Juss.: tirateima
Eugenia michelii Lam.: pitanga
Euphorbia pillulifera L.: corredeira
Ficus doliaria M.: gameleira
Gomphrena globosa L.: suspiro branco
Gossypium hirsutum L.: folha de algodão
Guettarda angelica Mart.: angélica
Hedychium coronarium Koen.: narciso branco
Helianthus annuus L.: girassol
Hybanthus ipecacuanha Bail.: purga do campo
Hyptis pectinata Poit.: folha de neve
Ionidium ipecacuanha Vent.: purga do campo
Ipomoea littoralis Boiss.: salsa da praia
Ipomoea pes-caprae Forsk.: salsa da praia

Jatropha curcas L.: pinhão branco
Jatropha gossypifolia Muell.: pinhão roxo
Jatropha oligandra Muell.: cansanção
Jatropha urens L.: cansanção
Kalanchoe brasiliensis: folha da Costa
Kanimia: abre caminhos
Kyllinga odorata Vahl.: capim santo
Lavandula spica L.: alfazema
Lavandula vera: alfazema
Leonurus sibiricus L.: cordão de São Francisco
Lepidum bonariense L.: mastruz
Lilium candidum L.: lirio branco
Lygodium polymorphum H.B.K.: sambambaia de caboclo
Marjorana hortensis: manjerona
Melissa officinalis L.: erva cidreira
Mentha pulegium L.: poejo
Mentha viridis L.: hortelã grosso
Miconia albicans: canela de velho
Mimosa nigra Hub.: jurema preta
Mirabilis jalapa L.: bonina
Momordica charantia L.: São Caetano
Monnieria trifolia L.: favaquinha de cobra
Musa: banana
Myristica fragrans Houtt.: noz moscada
Myrtus communis L.: murta
Ocimum basilicum L.: manjericão
Ocimum fluminensis V.: alfavaca
Ocimum guineensis Sch.: quioiô
Opuntia burbanki: palma
Opuntia dillenii Haw.: palma
Opuntia tuna Mill.: palma
Panicum crus-ardeae Willd.: nativo
Panicum elongatum Poir: nativo
Passiflora alata Ait.: maracujá
Passiflora bahiensis Klotzsch.: maracujá
Pavonia cancelata: jeribão
Peltodon radicans: folha santa
Petiveria alliacea L.: guiné
Petrea volubilis Jacq.: sapatinho de Nossa Senhora

Philodendron imbé Schott.: imbé
Pilea microphylla: brilhantina
Piper aduncum Vell.: tapa buraco
Piper eucaliptifolium Rudge: betis cheiroso
Pluchea quitoc D.C.: quitoco
Plumbago scandens L.: louco branco
Plumeria aurantia Lodd.: jasmin do Plário
Plumeria lutea R. & P.: jasmin do Plário
Polygala paniculata L.: barba de São Pedro
Polygonum acre H.B.K.: capiçoba
Pothos quadrangularis: folha de urubú
Psidium araçá Rad.: araçá de porco
Psidium cuneatum Camb.: araçá de porco
Psidium humile Vel.: araçá de porco
Renealmia brasiliensis Schum.: água de levante
Rhoeo discolor Hanc.: barquinho de Noé
Ricinus communis L.: folha de mamona
Rolandra argenta: vencetudo
Rosmarinus officinalis L.: alecrim
Ruta graveolens L.: arruda
Sambucus australis L.: sabugueiro
Sambucus nigra L.: sabugueiro
Sansevieria trifasciata laurentii: espada de Oxossi
Sansevieria zeylanica Willd.: espada de Ogun
Schinus molle L.: aroeira
Scoparia dulcis L.: vassourinha de Nossa Senhora
Sida acuta: vassourinha de relógio
Sida micrantha St Hil.: malva risco
Sida nudata Gand.: vassourinha de relógio
Sida rhombifolia Burm.: vassourinha de relógio
Solanum agrarium Sendt.: melancia da praia
Solanum balbisii Dum.: melancia da praia
Solanum paniculatum L.: jurubeba
Solanum pulverulentum: caiçara
Sparattanthelium botucudorum: arco de barris
Spondias cytherea: cajá
Stachys fluminensis: catinga de crioula
Struthanthus brasiliensis: erva de passarinho
Struthanthus vulgaris: erva de passarinho

Talinum patens Willd.: língua de vaca
Tapirira guianensis Aubl.: pau pombo
Urena lobata L.: malva risco
Vernonia bahiensis Toledo: aluman
Vernonia membranacia Gardn.: assapeixe branco
Viola ipecacuanha L.: purga do campo
Vismia brasiliensis Chois.: capianga
Wedelia paludosa D.C.: malmequer
Xanthium spinosum L.: juiz de paz
Xanthoxylum rhoifolium Lam.: espinho cheiroso
Xylopia: bejerecum
Zebrina pendula Schnitzl.: sapatinho de Nossa Senhora
Zinnia elegans Jacq.: canela de velho

APPENDIX THREE

PHONETIC TRANSCRIPTIONS

The International Phonetic Alphabet is used in all transcriptions.

Page

59: ɛˈʃɛ

125,

No. 1: sakolˈɛ sakolˈɛ ʒĩ: ʒĩ:

No. 2: saˈkwende kwa saˈkwende kwe

No. 3: sakaneˈne taˈte

No. 4: ʃɛ truˈa ʃɛ truˈa ʃɛ truˈa

126,

No. 6: oiˈju pɛ pɛ pɛ oiˈju pɛ pɛ pa oiˈju pɛ pɛ pɛ

127,

No. 6: ˈʃɛregede

No. 7: taˈta

No. 9: kebɛluˈʒa

ˈkwele ˈkwele ʒɔmbaˈla

128,

No. 11: ɛ taˈta ki: malemˈbe

No. 16: gɔˈro gɔˈsi:

na ʒo

No. 17: lɔkoˈja mwi:

129,

No. 23: ɛuˈwa ɛuˈwa ɛuˈwa ɛwˈwe

130,

No. 29: ˈkere keˈre

APPENDIX FOUR

THE QUESTION OF PAYMENT

A particularly significant feature in curing ritual is that of payment. All *curandeiros* interviewed mentioned how important it was that any ritual, however small, should be accompanied by payment. Their main reason for insisting on this was so that the ritual itself would retain its power, ritual without payment being considered worthless. This insistence is by no means primarily concerned with personal gain, though charges are levied in a very flexible manner and only in accordance with the economic standing of the patient. When I was investigating herbs, I had to pay informants a minimum sum (of approximately a halfpenny each) for each herb, a specimen of which was picked and given to me for examination. Again, it was considered in this instance that the herbs might lose their power if their secrets were passed on to me without payment.

Payment for ritual is never referred to as *pagamento* (payment), but as *troca* (exchange), and this terminology extends into the purchase of any article connected with ritual. Hence, for example, herbs in the market are not 'purchased' but 'exchanged', and people use the expression: *vou trocar ervas*, meaning, 'I am going *to buy* herbs.'[1]

I feel that this may be linked to the notion that evil may be avoided with a coin. The coin is not looked upon as payment but as a commodity used in order to barter. Evil is exchanged for money, and the word *trocar* survives to reinforce this notion.

It is common, particularly after a *sacudida* or *ebó* ritual, for the *curandeiro* to fumigate the money received in payment, and this reflects the idea that it has indeed been received in exchange for the evil force which has been removed. Moreover, the practice of keeping the payment for the *carregador do ebó* (known as *dinheiro do chão*) separate from that of the *curandeiro* reinforces this view in that the *carregador* has to transport to a suitable place all the substances contaminated in the course of the ritual. The *carregador* also lacks the protection afforded to the *curandeiro* by the nature of his office. The *dinheiro do chão* is left at the scene of the ritual, and either placed inside a small box on which the patient sits, or placed under his left foot (see above, page 116). This is akin to the instance in Greece recorded by Hardie (1923:166), in which the wise woman tramples a coin given to her in payment for curing the evil eye in case the evil has passed into it. Maclagan (1902 1st edn., 1972:30) mentions how the giving of a silver coin protects against the evil eye.

APPENDIX FIVE

Racial Composition of the Recôncavo

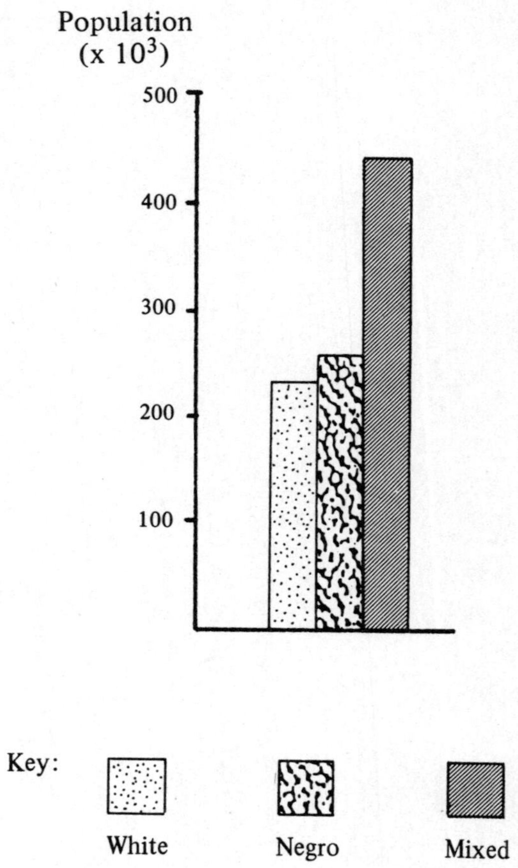

Reproduced by Henshall and Momsen (1974:222) from *Atlas Nacional do Brasil*, I.B.G.E., 1966, Plate V - 1

APPENDIX SIX

PERSONAL DETAILS CONCERNING INFORMANTS

Where possible, personal details include:

1. Sex
2. Age
3. Colour[1]
4. Family situation
5. Civil status
6. Own or husband's occupation
7. Economic status within own socio-economic group
8. Literacy
9. Whether or not a cult initiate and if so, status in cult
10. Dominant *orixá*[2]

Informants are listed below. Names are not given as the majority of informants specifically requested that their names should not be published.

I.1: Woman, 37. Dark *mulata*. Mother of large family. Married. Cleaner/washerwoman. Low economic status. Illiterate. Not cult initiate, but participated in *Candomblé* and spirit sessions as a medium. *Orixá* = Yansan.

I.2: Woman, 45. Black. Mother of large family. Separated.[3] Cleaner, partly supported by adult children in home. Low economic status. Literate. Initiate. *Mãe de santo*,[4] but with no *terreiro* of her own. *Orixá* = Oxossi.

I.3: Woman, 39. Black. Mother of three. Married. No present employment, formerly nursemaid to middle-class *Itaparicano* family. Low economic status. Illiterate. Initiate. *Mãe de santo* with small, poor *terreiro*. *Orixá* = Yansan.

I.4: Man, 40. Black. Father of three. Married. Small shopkeeper. Medium-low economic status. Literate. Initiate. Member of priestly hierarchy of *egun* (spirit of the dead) cult, Amoreiras, Itaparica. *Orixá* unknown.

I.5: Man, 38, Black. Father of two, brother of I.4. Married. Fisherman. Medium economic status. Literate. Initiate. Member of priestly hierarchy of *egun* cult. *Orixá* unknown.

I.6: Woman, 53. White. Mother of four. Married. No employment, husband seaman on mainland ferry service. Relatively prosperous economic status. Literate. Initiate. *Mãe de santo* with *terreiro* and house in Salinas (see *Map* 2) and *presidente* of spirit session held twice a month in Itaparica. *Orixá* = Oxun.

I.7: Woman, 30. White. Mother of three, daughter of I.6. Married. No employment, husband seaman on mainland ferry service. Shares maternal household. Literate. Initiate. *Mãe pequena*[6] of Salinas *terreiro* and *vice-presidente* of spirit session in Itaparica. *Orixá* = Yansan.

I.8: Woman, 40 approximately. Light *mulata*[7]. No family details obtainable. Member of semi-nomadic gipsy community moving about Recôncavo, camping for some months at Bom Despacho, Itaparica. Income mainly derived from selling cheap artefacts and telling fortunes of tourists on island and around Mercado Modêlo, Salvador. Very low economic status. Illiterate. Not an initiate.

C.1: Man, 51. Light *mulato*. Father of three. Married. No outside employment. Relatively prosperous economic status. Literate. Initiate. *Pai de santo* with own flourishing *terreiro*. *Orixá* = Xangô.

C.2: Man, 48. Dark *mulato*. Father of large family. Separated from legal wife, living with *mãe pequena* of *terreiro*. No outside employment. Medium-low economic status. Literate. Initiate. *Pai de santo* with *terreiro* in front room of own house, also used for spirit sessions, but under guidance of independent *presidente*. *Orixá* = Oxossi.

C.3: Woman, 44. Black. Mother of two. Separated. No outside employment. Relatively prosperous economic status. Literate. Initiate. *Mãe de santo* with highly commercialized *terreiro* (neon sign outside advertising consultancy services, etc.). *Orixá* = Martim Pescador.

C.4: Woman, 70. Black. Mother of large family, great-grandmother. Widow. No employment, supported by family. Low economic status. Illiterate. Initiate. *Mãe de santo* with own *terreiro*. *Orixá* unknown.

C.5: Man, 47. Dark *mulato*. No children. Married. No outside employment. Very low economic status. Illiterate. Initiate. *Pai de santo*, no *terreiro*. *Orixá* = Oxossi.

C.6: Woman, 49. Light *mulata*. Mother of large family. Married. No employment, husband railway company employee. Medium economic status. Literate. Initiate. Former *mãe de santo*, at present participant in *Candomblé* and spirit sessions. *Orixá* = Yemanjá.

C.7: Woman, 28. Black. Mother of four. Married. Cleaner/washerwoman, husband night-watchman. Low economic status. Literate. Initiate. *Filha de santo.*[8] *Orixá* = Yansan.

C.8: Man, 35. White. Father of four, husband of C.7. Night watchman. Low economic status. Literate. Initiate. *Ogã.*[9] *Orixá* = Oxalá.

C.9: Woman, 29. Black. Mother of three. Married. No outside employment. Husband labourer. Low economic status. Illiterate. Initiate. One of youngest *mães de santo*, own *terreiro*. *Orixá* = Ogun.

C.10: Man, 59. Black. Unmarried. Employee in small commercial enterprise. Relatively prosperous economic status. Literate. Initiate. *Pai de santo*, own *terriero*, Malé cult. *Orixá* unknown.

C.11: Man, 19. Light *mulato*. Unmarried. No employment. Literate. Initiate. Planning to set up own *terreiro* (completed successfully, 1975). *Orixá* = Oxossi.

C.12: Woman, 55. Dark *mulata*. Mother of large family. Married. No outside employment, husband's occupation unknown. Relatively prosperous economic status. Semi-literate. Initiate. *Mãe de santo*, newly built *terreiro* opened 1974. *Orixá* = Ogun.

C.13: Man, 67. White. No children. Married. Retired. Medium economic status. Literate. Not cult initiate.

C.14: Woman, 61. Black. No family details obtainable. Small shopkeeper. Low economic status. Illiterate. Not cult initiate, but participant in *Candomblé*. *Orixá* unknown.

C.15: Woman, 41. Dark *mulata*. Mother of large family. Separated. Cigar-roller in tobacco factory. Low economic status. Illiterate. Initiate. *Filha de santo*. *Orixá* = Omolú.

S.1: Woman, 57. Black. Mother of large family. Widow. Washerwoman employed in private house. Low economic status, but supported by employers. Illiterate. Not cult initiate, but participant in *Candomblé*.

S.2: Woman, approximately 45–55. Black. Mother (size of family not known). Married. No outside employment, husband's occupation not known. Relatively prosperous economic situation. Literate. Initiate. *Mãe de santo* with flourishing *terreiro*, one of oldest established and best-known in Salvador. *Orixá* = Yansan.

S.3: Woman, 67. Dark *mulata*. Size of family not known. Separated. No details of employment known. Low economic status. Illiterate. Initiate. *Mãe pequena* in S.2's *terreiro*. *Orixá* unknown.

S.4: Man, 56. Light *mulato*. Size of family unknown. Married. No outside employment. Low economic status. Literate. Initiate. *Pai de santo* with own *terreiro* in poor suburb of city. *Orixá* = Oxossi.

S.5: Woman, 52. Light *mulata*. Unmarried. Teacher in primary school. High economic status. Not cult initiate but participant in spirit sessions.

S.6: Woman, 75. Dark *mulata*. Unmarried. Stallholder (herb seller) in Mercado Modêlo. Low economic status. Literate. Not initiate, but participant in *Candomblé*. *Orixá* = Oxun.

S.7: Boy, 16. Dark *mulato*. Unmarried. Stallholder (herb seller) in Mercado Santa Bárbara. Medium-low economic status. Literate. Not initiate, but participant in *Candomblé*. *Orixá* unknown.

S.8: Man, 26. Light *mulato*. Father of one. Separated. Stallholder in Mercado Santa Bárbara. Low economic status. Literate. Initiate. *Ogã*. *Orixá* = Omolú.

S.9: Man, 35. Black. Father of large family. Married. Street herb-seller. Low economic status. Illiterate. Not cult initiate, but participant in *Candomblé*. *Orixá* = Oxalá.

S.10: Woman, 31. Dark *mulata*. Mother of two. Widow. Stallholder in Mercado Santa Bárbara. Low economic status. Literate. Initiate. *Filha de santo*. *Orixá* = Yemanjá.

P.1: Man, 45. Light *mulato*.[10] Family size unknown. Married. Chief of Pataxó tribe living on reservation near Porto Seguro in south of state of Bahia. Economic status within reservation unknown. Illiterate. No connection with *Candomblé*.

R.1: Woman, 60 approximately. Black. Unwilling to disclose family details. Separated. No outside employment. High economic status. Literate. Initiate. *Mãe de santo* presiding over extremely flourishing *terreiro* on outskirts of Rio de Janeiro. *Orixá* = Exú.

G.1: Woman, 38. White. Mother of five. Married. No employment, husband fisherman. Low economic status. Literate.

G.2: Man, 55. White. Father of large family. Married. Agricultural worker. Medium economic status. Literate.

GLOSSARY

Abaluayé: See Omolú
abó: Ritual bath
abrir (*abre*) *caminhos:* Literally 'open the ways'; resolve difficulties
acaçá: Balls of ground maize cooked in water and wrapped in banana leaves
acarajé: A fried maize cake often served with a hot, spicy sauce, and sold in the street
afastar: To repel; to drive away
alguidar: Earthenware bowl in which the *ebó* is placed
alho macho/fêmeo: Male and female garlic, male garlic being long and thin and female garlic squat and rounded
amasi: Ritual bath
ar: Ill wind
ar de morto: Rather akin to *mofina de morto*, but the *ar de morto* is never seen. The dead person's spirit lingers near the living and distracts them
atotó Baba: The cry of salutation for Omolú
atraer: To attract

Babá: Father. Term of affection for Omolú
babalorixá: A *pai de santo* (q.v.)
banho: Ritual bath. Also known as *banho de cheiro*
banho de descarga/discarrego: A ritual bath
banho de desenvolvimento: A ritual bath
bori: A ritual that takes place in the cult house involving the sacrifice of an animal, the blood of which must be drunk by the person on whom the *bori* is being performed. For further details, see page 18
breve: Amulet. See Chapter IX
brincadeira: Game, from *brincar*, to jump
búzios: Cowrie shells

caboclo: Indian spirit
cachaça: Sugar-cane brandy
camarinha: Literally 'small room'. The room in the cult house where initiation takes place. Also known as *ile orixá*

Candomblé: African religion in Bahia. See particularly Chapter III
Candomblé de caboclo: For a full definition of this term see pages 18–20
carregador (*do ebó*): The person who carries away the *ebó* and dumps it in a suitable place
consulta: Consultation between a person and a *pai/mãe de santo*
contas: Beads worn by cult initiates
copo de vidência: A glass of water used for divination in a spirit session
de corpo limpo: Ritually clean body, cf. *corpo sujo*
de corpo sujo: Ritually soiled body, cf. *corpo limpo*
corrente: Literally 'current', but see page 10 and page 103 n. 41
curandeirismo: Folk medicine, curing
curandeiro: One who practises *curandeirismo*, a curer

degredado: Criminal, religious or political exile
despacho da porta: For a description of this ritual, see pages 66–7
desquitado/a: One who is separated
desquite: Legal separation of man and wife
dinheiro do chão: Floor money. Money left on the floor during an *ebó* ritual in payment of the *carregador do ebó*'s services

ebó: For the meaning of this word, see Chapter XI *passim*
egun: Spirit of the dead
encorrentar: Literally 'to pass a current', but see page 103 n. 41
engenho: Sugar plantation and mill
epa hei: A cry of salutation for Yansan
eré: Semi-trance; the intermediate stage between the normal and the ecstatic state; a state of calm, childish ecstasy
espírito: Spirit
Exú: One of the *orixás*. Syncretized with the devil. The god of mischief. The term Exú may also mean an evil spirit
Exú é: The cry of salutation for Exú

fechar o corpo: To close/seal the body against evil influences
figa: An amulet carved in the shape of a clenched fist with the thumb clasped between the fore and middle fingers
filho(*a*) *de santo*: Initiated and fully participant male or female cult member. Literally 'son (or daughter) of the saints'
fluído: Literally 'fluid transmitted by a spirit'
fulano: Roughly equivalent to 'so-and-so'

guía: Guide

Ibeji: Orixás (the twins). Syncretized with Cosmas and Damian. They are the patrons of all children

ile orixá: See *camarinha*

influência ruim: Bad/evil influence that may contribute to illness

ingolosí: Formal prayers sung at specific times during the day in the cult house. Also sung during the preparation of *pemba*

invidia: Envy

irmão de luz: Literally 'spirit of light', i.e. one who is free from all evil

kawó Xangôkabiyesi le: The cry of salutation for Xangô

limpar: To clean; cleanse

limpeza (de corpo): Cleansing (of the body), but see also *ebó*

limpeza das águas: Cleansing by the waters. Part of the *ebó* ritual

limpeza dos astros: Cleansing by the stars. Part of the *ebó* ritual

Macumba: Name of an African religion in the south of Brazil (particularly in Rio de Janeiro and São Paulo)

mãe de santo: A high priestess in the *Candomblé* cult. Literally 'mother of the saints'

mãe pequena: Assistant to the *mãe de santo*

malembe: Mercy

maracá: Gourd rattle

massapé: Type of soil in the Recôncavo which is particularly suited to the cultivation of sugar and tobacco

mau de olho: Evil eye

mau olhado: Evil eye

milho: Maize

mofina/mofina de morto: The spirit of a dead person who haunts the living

moléstia do ar: Illness brought by the ill wind

mulato(a): The meaning of this term in the context of the present study is given on page 163 n. 1

Nagô: The common language of the original Yoruba-speaking tribes in Africa

Naná: One of the *orixás*. Syncretized with Saint Anne. The old matriarch of the Yoruba pantheon of deities

Obaluayé: See Omolú
obi: A ritual that takes place in the cult house. An *obi* nut is cut into four sections and placed on the scalp. For further details, see page 18
obrigação: Literally 'obligation'. The word is used to refer to any sacrifice or offering to the *orixás*
oferenda aos caboclos: Offering to the *caboclos*. Part of the *ebó* ritual
ogã: Male holder of post of responsibility within the *terreiro*
Ogun: One of the *orixás*. Syncretized with Saint Anthony. The god of war
Ogun ye: The cry of salutation for Ogun
olhado: Evil eye
olho grosso: Evil eye
olho mal (*mau*): Evil eye
Olorun: One of the *orixás*. Syncretized with God the Father
Omolú: One of the *orixás*. Syncretized with Saints Lazarus and Roche. The god of disease, particularly smallpox. Also known as Obaluayé and Abaluayé
orixá: A god. The god to whom a person may be dedicated within the terms of the *Candomblé* religion
otá: Stones that represent the *orixás*. They are kept in the *pejí*
Oxalá: One of the *orixás*. Syncretized with Jesus Christ
Oxossi: One of the *orixás*. Syncretized with Saint George. The god of the hunt
Oxun: One of the *orixás*. Syncretized with the Virgin Mary. The goddess of fresh water and fertility
oya: A cry of salutation for Yansan. It is also one of her other names

pade de Exú: Offering made to Exú at the beginning of most rituals. Also known as *despacho de Exú*
pagé: Shaman
pai de santo: A high priest in the *Candomblé* cult. Literally 'father of the saints'
Pará: Name of an African religion in Porto Alegre
passe; dar um passe: For the meaning of this term, see page 103 n. 42
patuá: Amulet. See Chapter IX
pejí: Sanctuary in the cult house
pemba/pemba preparada: A white powder made from crushed dried herbs. See Chapter VIII
pemba de Exú, pemba preta: A black powder used for evil purposes. See Chapter VIII

ponto riscado: Cabbalistic sign usually drawn with *pemba*
presidente: President

quebranto(e): Overlooking
queda de orixá: Literally 'fall of the *orixá*'. The term refers to the moment when a person is possessed by his *orixá* for the first time

rezar: To pray while brushing a sprig of leaves over the affected area. See Chapter X

sacudida: A ritual beating with specific herbs. See Chapter V
santo: Saint
seita: Sect
senhor de engenho: Sugar-plantation owner
Sertão: Interior hinterland that stretches from Bahia northwards to Ceará
sessão espírita: *Séance*, spirit session

terreiro: Cult house
trabalho: Work, but see *ebó*
Umbanda: Religion in the south of Brazil, particularly Rio de Janeiro and São Paulo
urubú: A large black bird that feeds on carrion—*Cathartes foetens*, C. (C.A.)

vento mal: Ill wind

Xangô: Name of an African religion in Recife. Also one of the *orixás*. Syncretized with Saint Jerome. Controls thunder

Yansan: One of the *orixás*. Syncretized with Saint Barbara. Goddess of the thunderbolt
Yemanjá: One of the *orixás*. Syncretized with the Virgin Mary. The goddess of salt water and fertility

NOTES AND REFERENCES

(For list of abbreviations, see Bibliography, page 200)

PREFACE

1. The interior hinterland. The term *sertão* covers an enormous area of the north-eastern interior, from Bahia to Ceará.
2. People in higher socio-economic groups were found to be unwilling to admit any connection with *curandeirismo* or *Candomblé* and displayed a dismissive or disapproving attitude, even though, on occasions, they were known to be, or to have been, participants in associated rituals.
3. See, for example, Appendix One, which lists the herbs and their uses.

CHAPTER I. THE RECÔNCAVO: ITS GEOGRAPHY, HISTORY AND PEOPLE

1. Statistics taken from the *Investors Chronicle*, London, 4 July 1975.
2. Pierson 1967:10.
3. Freyre dedicates a whole volume to this region: see Freyre 1946.
4. Henshall and Momsen 1974:66, on whom I draw for much of the information in this section.
5. Henshall and Momsen 1974:115–16 (figures for 1970).
6. See Freyre 1946, esp. pp. 24, 43, 175.
7. *Pau-Brasil*, a dyewood with a rich red hue.
8. Henshall and Momsen 1974:33.
9. See below, pages 5–6.
10. Pierson 1967:7.
11. Henshall and Momsen 1974:34.
12. Henshall and Momsen 1974:11, 15.
13. For a fuller discussion of these survivals and contributions, see Freyre 1946:81–184; Azevedo 1969:57–152; Pierson 1967:111–37; Henshall and Momsen 1974:9–32; Ott 1955:18–34.
14. This pattern was somewhat modified, however, in the Recôncavo, as Henshall and Momsen point out (1974:37), by the concentration on tobacco and diversification into the produce of food crops for commercial markets.

15. See Appendix Five.

Chapter II. The Religious Background: Indian, African and European Influences

1. Ott 1955:I, 18ff., 31.
2. For a fuller discussion of Tupi religions, see Métraux I and II, 1928; Freyre 1946:81ff.; Radin 1942:75ff.
3. Ribeiro 1970:55–69; Wilson 1975:206–16.
4. Freyre 1946:107.
5. Freyre 1946:138.
6. Ramos 1946:281. Ott (1955:I, 54) estimates that there were 10,000 African slaves in Lisbon during the sixteenth century.
7. Ott 1955:I, 58.
8. Ramos 1946:275.
9. Ramos 1946:282; Pierson 1967:71–2.
10. Nagô as a 'general language' must not be confused with the earlier *língua geral* imposed by the Jesuits to facilitate communication between Indians who spoke different Tupi dialects and the first Portuguese colonizers. See Freyre 1946:39, 42, 107.
11. Verger 1957:16; Ramos 1946:268.
12. Ott 1955:I, 59.
13. Ramos 1946:267–8.
14. Pierson 1967:33–4.
15. Verger 1957:17–18.
16. Ott 1955:I, 60ff.
17. Verger 1957:18.
18. Burton 1869:I, 270.
19. Pierson 1967:335, 346.
20. Pierson 1967:73; Koster 1816:I, 229.
21. Ramos 1946:317; see also Etienne 1909.
22. Southey 1810:II, 674.
23. Ott 1955:I, 46ff.
24. Ott 1955:I, 50–51.
25. See esp. Freyre 1946:254ff.; Castillo de Lucas 1951, 1958, 1963; Lima Carneiro and Pires de Lima 1943; Dias 1944; Vasconcellos 1882, 1892, 1906, 1925, 1958, 1960; Bouza Brey 1949; Lis Quibén 1945, 1949; Rodriguez López 1895; Barriola 1952.
26. Henshall and Momsen 1974:232, 234.

27. Henshall and Momsen 1974:234.
28. The terms Spiritism and Spiritualism tend to be used arbitrarily by writers in English, and there is no clearcut distinction between them (O.E.D.). I have chosen to use the term Spiritism since it is closest to Rivail's use of the French term *Spiritisme* and the Brazilian *Espiritismo*.
29. See esp. Rivail 1857 and 1864.
30. For general studies on Spiritism, with particular reference to Brazil, see Wilson 1975:117–20; McGregor 1966; St Clair 1971.
31. See also below, page 103 n. 41.
32. Wilson 1975:119.
33. St Clair (1971: opposite 161) gives an illustration.

Chapter III. The Persistence and Development of African Religions

1. See Freyre 1946:370–71, where it is stated how the African readily embraced baptism so as to be socially equal to his fellow slaves. The unbaptized (pagan) slave was considered inferior.
2. Pierson 1967:94ff.; Freyre 1946:472.
3. See esp. *A Tarde* (Bahia), 9 December, 1935, 8 May, 1936, 10 June, 1937.
4. Gallet 1934:57.
5. Olga de Alakêto was referred to in the Bahia press during her official visit to Nigeria in 1974 as *Princesa* Dona Olga de Alakêto.
6. For general studies on *Candomblé*, see esp. Bastide 1961; Verger 1957; Carneiro 1961; Rodrigues 1935.
7. See Ribeiro 1952. *Xangô* is also the name given to the cult in Trinidad; see Simpson 1962.
8. The precise origin and meaning of *Pará* is unclear. It may derive from Elebara, the god of mischief in the south of Brazil. See Herskovits 1943:503 n. 8.
9. For general studies on *Macumba* and *Umbanda*, see esp. McGregor 1966; St Clair 1971.
10. The problem of relationships between Catholicism and other religions in Brazil is a complex one, and so these comments are restricted to the Recôncavo of Bahia.
11. The Nagô spoken in traditional cult houses in Brazil has remained very conservative, mainly because it tends to be spoken only during specific rituals, and it contains many archaisms when compared with

the Yoruba currently spoken in Nigeria. Brazilian *Candomblé* priests from traditional cult houses are extremely proud of being able to converse freely in the Yoruba language when in Africa. It is stressed that this knowledge of Yoruba is restricted to traditional houses.

12. See Carneiro 1961:17–18; Bastide 1961:17.
13. For a discussion of the semantic links between jumping, play and religious ritual in other languages, see Huizinga 1971:33–51.
14. Verger 1957:403.
15. Verger 1957:209.
16. A minor *orixá* with little devotional following in Brazil nowadays.
17. Bastide 1961:249–50.
18. cf. Wallis Budge (1928:28), who says of the Egyptians: 'Every member of the body of a living man was protected by a god, and the *Book of the Dead* (Chapter XLII) shows us that the members of a dead man were believed to be protected in the same way.' cf. also the Catholic idea of patron saints.
19. For the *eré*, see Bastide 1961:253ff.; Simpson 1962:1211–12; Herskovits 1948:9.
20. The Ibeji have become syncretized with the Catholic 'twins', Cosmas and Damian. They are patrons of all children.
21. This is particularly the case with *abó*, which is a mixture kept for a long time and hence acquires a most distinctive rotten smell. See below, pages 54–57.
22. For *obi*, see Querino 1955:60–63; Rodrigues 1935:81. For *bori*, see Carneiro 1961:106; Verger 1957:80–95.
23. The souls of the dead are believed to travel west, hence the early slaves found Itaparica to be an ideal location for the *egun* cult. This cult is still largely unknown, partly because of its isolation (the cult house is on a remote hilltop), and partly because the male priests who officiate appear to be mainly members of the same family and are extremely wary of allowing outsiders to attend rituals.
24. Reference is made particularly to the following *seitas*: Opo Afonjá; Olga de Alakêto; Meninina de Gantois (Salvador); Albertino (Cachoeira); Egun (Amoreiras, Itaparica).
25. There was even a serious attempt at this time to establish Tupi Guarani as the language of the Brazilian intellectual.
26. Binon Cossard 1970:154–5.
27. For a brief description of *Candomblé de caboclo*, see Querino 1938:125–7 and Ramos 1940:159–64.

28. This is not the case in Rio de Janeiro, where a lot of Tupi can be identified in the incantations and in the ritual language in general (R.1).
29. For further information concerning Aruanda, see Câmara Cascudo 1965:90–95.
30. Binon Cossard 1970:150, 154.
31. Ramos 1940:161. See also *ibid.*:165–8 for a fairly comprehensive list of Catholic saints with their African/*caboclo* counterparts.
32. On one occasion I.1 attributed accidentally bumping her head to an *influência ruim* (bad influence) despite the fact that all the ill-effects of the accident disappeared within twenty-four hours.
33. The differences and similarities between the *mau de olho* and *moléstia do ar* are somewhat more involved than this, however, and these are dealt with in greater detail below. See pages 100 and 106–9.
34. See esp. Lévy-Bruhl 1926; Ramos 1940:213; Rodrigues 1935:92–7; Blache 1963:30; Machado Filho 1964:41–2; Bastide 1950:7; Campos 1967:19–20; Magalhães 1966:8–9; Maynard Araújo 1961:55, 1958: 64; MacLean 1974:139.

Chapter IV. Herbs

1. 'Herbs' is here intended as a generic term to include leaves, roots, nuts, seeds, fruits, etc.
2. See esp. Bastide 1961:156, where an informant is quoted as saying, *Todo o segrêdo do candomblé reside em suas ervas* ('the whole secret of *Candomblé* lies in its herbs'); Verger 1957:229–31.
3. Bastide 1961:156.
4. Also noted by Binon Cossard 1970:173.
5. Such flexibility is not shown, however, in traditional *seitas*.
6. The post-fix *de caboclo* does not always imply that the plant belongs to a *caboclo* spirit. cf. *capim de caboclo*, which belongs to Yansan and Oxossi.
7. Also observed by Menezes 1949:183; Ramos 1940:194, who gives *pipi* as a variant; *pipi* is also given by Gomes 1809 1st edn. 1972:29 and Hoehne 1939:112–13.
8. Pardal 1937:173.
9. Quoted by Câmara Cascudo 1951:83.
10. Correa 1969:I, 180; Gifford 1958:74–6, also stresses the historical importance of rue.

11. Debret n.d.: II, plate 11.
12. Andrade 1963:229.
13. There are important exceptions, however, which will be pointed out later. See below, page 43–4.
14. An informant (I.6) once described Yansan as *uma mulher macha* ('a manly woman').
15. Yansan carries a sword and her colour is red.
16. *Rezar* means literally 'to pray'. The *curandeiro* says a prayer or charm while lightly brushing leaves over the patient's body. See Chapter X below.
17. cf. Barroso 1923:295–6, who mentions how plants in the hot pepper family wilt and dry up completely if a victim of the evil eye looks at them.
18. See also Bastide 1961:158, 1950:9. However, Vogel 1970:51, quoting Bricknell, tells of North American Indians who cultivated herb gardens to guarantee a ready supply.
19. This aspect of curing is discussed in greater detail below. See pages 66–71.
20. cf. Vogel 1970:29, who mentions how medicine men in North America performed ceremonies to make their herbs powerful.
21. cf. Douglas 1970:20, who mentions how taboos in the past often took the form of rules of uncleanness.
22. Bastide 1961:158–9; Krappe (1962:192–3) gives rhymes that accompanied the picking of healing herbs in Europe to increase their efficacy.
23. That the intention should be perfectly clear in the mind of the picker is a medieval feature too. See Thorndike 1947:I, 79.
24. A white powder made from crushed dried herbs. See below, Chapter VIII.
25. McKenzie 1927:189. cf. Cardinall n.d.:23, who points out how in Africa on the Gold Coast, people blow ash towards the new moon because they fear that an increase in the power of the moon would bring about a decrease in their own strength.
26. Magalhães 1966:151.
27. Pliny II:CII, 349. See also Pettigrew 1844:21; Magalhães 1966:12–14. In medieval theory, the balance of humours in the human body was believed to change in accordance with the phases of the moon. See Curry 1960:13–14. Such beliefs were still being expounded in the early eighteenth century by Richard Mead, vice-president of the

Royal Society, who wrote in 1708 a *Discourse concerning the Action of the Sun and Moon on Animal Bodies; and the Influence which This may have in many Diseases.*

28. Blache 1963:35; Castillo de Lucas 1958–132; Taboada 1952:617–22.
29. McKenzie 1927:154. The feast of St John falls in the middle of Brazilian winter, but it has retained the special significance the old Midsummer Day still has in Europe.
30. On this point, see Vogel 1970:137, who points out how certain North American Indians considered some herbs to be at maximum strength only when collected in a certain brief season. See also Burton 1628:366, who quotes Bassardus Viscontinus as saying St John's wort gathered on a Friday about the full moon in July will be at its most powerful in combating melancholy and driving away spirits.
31. Friday is the day set aside for the worship of Oxalá. The original African week was divided into four days set aside in honour of the four elements (earth, air, water and fire), the four cardinal points, and, by extension, the deities who presided over them. Some redistribution of days of worship to conform with the European calendar was therefore necessary when the Africans arrived in Brazil. Days set aside for certain *orixás* and practices do not therefore correspond exactly to those currently observed in Africa. For a further discussion of this point, see Bastide 1961:120–28. It is probable that Friday was set aside for Oxalá (syncretized with Jesus Christ) because it was on that day that Christ died.
32. In certain rural areas of Britain, the custom still survives of planting parsley seeds on Good Friday.
33. Taboada (1947:123) quotes the following verse illustrating the way twelve o'clock is associated with ill-fortune:

   Between twelve and one
   Walks ill fortune;
   Between one and two
   Walks the Mother of God.

   Midnight has always been considered to be a rather dangerous time, as the English expression 'witching hour' bears witness. See also Binon Cossard (1970:219), who mentions that it is dangerous for the initiate to leave the cult house at midnight, 6 a.m. and midday. These times are known popularly in Brazil as *as horas abertas* ('open hours', i.e. open to evil influence).

34. Dawson 1935:35–6; McKenzie 1927:152. The concept of linking a herb to a planet was developed principally by Paracelsus in the sixteenth century and expanded in Europe by herbalists such as Nicholas Culpeper who based their theories on ancient Babylonian and Egyptian astrology. Culpeper (1653 1st edn. 1850:V) gives precise instructions in the epistle to his *The Complete Herbal* as to how diseases may be cured by herbs:

'The Herbs, Plants &c. are now in the book appropriated to their proper planets. Therefore,

'First, Consider what planet causeth the disease; that thou mayest find it in my aforesaid Judgment of Diseases.

'Secondly, Consider what part of the body is afflicted by the disease, and whether it lies in the flesh, or blood, or bones, or ventricles.

'Thirdly, Consider by what planet the afflicted part of the body is governed: that my Judgment of Diseases will inform you also.

'Fourthly, You may oppose diseases by Herbs of the planet, opposite to the planet that causes them: as diseases of *Jupiter* by herbs of *Mercury*, and the contrary; diseases of the *Luminaries* by the herbs of *Saturn*, and the contrary; diseases of *Mars* by herbs of *Venus*, and the contrary.

'Fifthly, There is a way to cure diseases sometimes by *Sympathy*, and so every planet cures his own disease; as the *Sun* and *Moon* by their Herbs cure the Eyes, *Saturn* the Spleen, *Jupiter* the Liver, *Mars* the Gall and diseases of choler, and *Venus* diseases in the instruments of Generation.'

It is likely that the close resemblance between Yoruba and medieval European herbal practice stems mainly from a common Babylonian and Egyptian source. Ideas from this source were widely diffused throughout the ancient world. Certainly African religions in Brazil display numerous traits characteristic of ancient Egypt and subsequently of Islam. In Egypt, for example, the connection between herbs and the gods was very close (see Wallis Budge 1928:24). For the principal contributions of ancient Egypt to medieval and Renaissance European herbal theory, see esp. Wallis Budge 1913 and 1928.

35. cf. Culpeper 1653 1st edn 1850:201; Black 1883:125–6, 129; Pettigrew 1844:19–20.

Chapter V. The Sacudida (Ritual Beating)

1. Freyre 1946:150–51, who even goes on to suggest that a number of Brazilian children's games reflect this practice of flagellation today.
2. Parrinder 1969:115, who should be consulted for more information on the *egun* and similar cults in Africa (pp. *ibid.*:115–36). See also Simpson 1962:1212; Verger 1957:507–10. For the *egun* cult in Brazil, see Lima 1946:5–14; Binon Cossard 1970:244ff.; Bastide 1961:167–80.
3. This point is dealt with at greater length on page 100.
4. See Chapter X.
5. This is known as the *pade de Exú*, and is adequately accounted for in myths. See Verger 1957:110–11; Bastide 1961:217–19; Carneiro 1961:80–83. The food offering usually consists of three small dishes of manioc flour mixed with *dendê* oil, *cachaça* (sugar-cane brandy) and water respectively.
6. Verger 1957:248–9, 256–69 (Verger's orthography).
7. *Oya* is the cry of salutation for Yansan. It is also one of her other names. See Verger 1957:402ff.
8. Such a spirit is called *ar de morto*, and will be dealt with later at greater length. See page 108.
9. Such reactions among the *orixás* are typical and occur frequently in myths. Also, whenever two protagonists in the same myth take possession of their mediums, they re-enact their mutual animosity or affection according to myth. Note particularly the jealousy that exists between Oxun and Obá, both wives of Xangô, who fight each other when they take possession of their mediums. See above, page 15.
10. The cry of salutation for Ogun.

Chapter VI. Fumigation

1. Câmara Cascudo 1962:II, 406; Lima 1959:9.
2. Castillo de Lucas 1963:306–7.
3. This later became syncretized with St John's feast day. See above, p. 28.
4. Castillo de Lucas 1963:305–6.
5. Maynard Araújo 1958:155. The Inca in Peru believed that direct contact with fire would destroy any evil force causing illness, and

during the *citua* festival people would beat each other with fire torches to rid themselves of disease. See Pardal 1937:156.

6. See Chapter X.
7. Bastide 1961:45; Binon Cossard 1970:190.
8. João do Rio 1906:22–3.
9. See Bouisson 1960:217.
10. Verger 1957:305.
11. For more information about the sacred character of the smith and his trade, and the identification of the craft of the smith with shamanism, healing, incantations, etc., see Eliade 1962.
12. Frobenius 1973:246.
13. Lévi-Strauss 1973:246.
14. Reichel-Dolmatoff 1971:194. On this point, see also Lévi-Strauss 1970.
15. Karsten 1926:381–2.
16. Stade 1874:147. See also Câmara Cascudo 1962:I, 271–2, 371–2.
17. Métraux 1946:530.
18. Menezes 1957:95–6.
19. Andrade 1963:214; Murphy and Murphy 1974:84.
20. Anon. (1) 1750:45–6 divides substances for fumigation into two similar categories.
21. Harper 1964:182–3.
22. See also Maynard Araújo 1961:149.
23. This is a very common cure for a minor stroke that results in partial paralysis (included under *moléstia do ar*, see below, pages 106–8) the idea behind it being to jerk the patient back to normality with a bitter brew.
24. The ferry service from the mainland began some fifteen years ago.
25. See, in particular, Waite 1911; Thorndike 1947; Summers 1945: 116–59.
26. They are well known as publications on occult rituals throughout the world in many languages, and their popularity today in Brazil is based mainly on the fact that they are the standard handbooks for anyone interested in performing such rituals. Legends have grown up around their use (such as the fairly common belief that, if a man reads one of them from cover to cover, he is bound to commit suicide), and there is usually a copy of one or both of them in the average *curandeiro*'s house. For details on Saint Cyprian, see Thorndike 1947:I, 428–32; Wallis Budge 1930:476; Wingate 1930; Summers 1945:122.

27. Fifteen different varieties were sold on average each day by each of five stalls picked at random in the Mercado Santa Barbara and the Mercado Modêlo (Salvador).
28. Ramos 1940:218–19 gives the names of some fumigators sold in Niterói. See also Castillo de Lucas 1958, who gives an illustration of a marketed variety of fumigator acquired in Bahia (*ibid.*: 54).
29. Binon Cossard 1970:290.
30. See also Ramos 1940:345, and Bastide 1961:191 n. 99.
31. See above, page 33.
32. Verger 1957:292.
33. See esp. Ramos (1940:320–23), who quotes incidents that appeared in the *Diario da Noite* (Rio de Janeiro), 12 October 1938, and in *A Tarde* (Bahia), 2 January 1931. In 1974, during the installation of a sewer outlet at Rio Vermelho beach (Salvador), unusually high seas delayed work for some months and a number of workers' lives were lost. Local people unanimously declared that Yemanjá was angered at the prospect of a sewer outlet being constructed on a beach that has traditionally been reserved for her worship by fishermen and others, especially on her two major feast days of the year (2 February and 8 December). See Verger 1957:293; Ramos 1940:306; Tavares n.d.:65ff. See also Hole 1967:184–6 for further details concerning the role of ancient sea gods.
34. See, for example, in Appendix One: *alfazema; folha de laranja da terra; malva risco.*
35. See also Lima 1946:101.
36. Mentioned by Valle 1963:596.
37. Valle *ibid.*
38. Vasconcellos 1882:121.

Chapter VII. Ritual Baths

1. Menezes 1957:44. This custom is based not so much on the notion that the river's flow would, according to the principles of 'sympathetic magic', ease the birth of the child, as on the idea that all men are connected with paradise by means of rivers, which are looked upon as being umbilical cords. The human mother assumes the role of the earth mother by giving birth on the banks of a river. On this point, see Reichel Dolmatoff 1971:57.
2. de Léry 1972:210.

3. Métraux and Baldus 1946:442.
4. Oberg 1953:102.
5. Menezes 1957:44.
6. Fundação Nacional do Indio, a government Indian protection foundation.
7. Karsten 1926:482.
8. Harper 1964:153. Harper's article is discussed by Douglas 1970.
9. For the Moslem influence among the African peoples of Brazil, see Rodrigues 1935:28–33.
10. See Bascom 1950, and Bastide 1961:90–91. See also Carneiro 1961: 105–6 for the annual rite of purification known as *água de Oxalá* (Oxalá's water).
11. Eliade 1962:55 stresses the importance of ritual purity when entering into the presence of the sacred. See also Anon. 1750:126.
12. Andrade 1963:221–2.
13. See Douglas 1970, esp. pp. 46–7.
14. Krappe 1962:296.
15. See also Maynard Araújo 1961:153.
16. This is a glass of water used for divination. See below, page 131.
17. A corruption of the word *descarregamento* (unburdening).
18. Câmara Cascudo 1962:I, 93.
19. Anon. (1) 1750:42 recommends the exorcizer to do as follows: 'Il faut qu'il se purifie avec l'eau exorcisée depuis le sommet de la tête jusques aux pieds . . . '
20. It may also be followed by the application of *pemba*. See next chapter.
21. Harper 1964:156.
22. It is worth noting that there is a herb called *abre caminhos* which belongs to Ogun.
23. See above, page 43.
24. The words are Yoruba, adopted by the *Candomblé de caboclo* followers.
25. Binon Cossard 1970:179, 181.
26. For *obi* and *bori*, see above, page 18.
27. Ramos 1940:66.
28. Câmara Cascudo 1951:93. Rodrigues (1900:56–7) describes it as 'des infusions de plantes qui jouissent les propriétés très stimulantes et qui sont considérées comme sacrées'.
29. Bascom (1950:66) records a similar procedure in Cuba.
30. Bascom 1950:65.
31. For the use of the *obi* in divination, see Simpson 1962: 1208–9.

32. cf. Binon Cossard 1970:181.
33. Bastide 1961:154.
34. Binon Cossard 1970:249.

Chapter VIII. Pemba (Ritual Powder)

1. Transcribed by Ribeiro and given by Bastide 1961: 236–7.
2. Bastide 1973:256.
3. The analyses of substances given in this chapter are based on infra-red spectroscopy conducted by the Department of Chemistry of the University of St Andrews. This corresponds to Binon Cossard's findings (1970:353): '... poudre blanche à base de kaolin'.
4. I am informed by L. Hoggarth of the C.L.A.L.S., St Andrews, that a similar sexual distinction is made by the Quechua in Cuzco, Peru, with regard to different mineral substances that make up the *hampi*. cf. Pardal 1937:163. See Lira (1946: 83–4), who describes *siwaryu* as: 'unos minerales en polvo que se consigue donde hay lagos. Es de dos clases: macho y hembra (orkkówan, chináwan) ... La gente recoge a la quita quita, porque tienen fé que es un gran remedio, principalmente para el susto ...' See also Lira (1960:41), where he mentions that these powders are to be found in twelve different colours.
5. Binon Cossard 1970:245, 249.
6. cf. Ramos 1941:134: 'Utilizam-se ainda os macumbeiros do Rio de Janeiro da pemba, ou giz para riscar um ponto e traçar symbolos dos "santos"...'
7. Its origins are fundamentally Judaic. See Spence 1920:240–42, and esp. Danzel 1947:157ff.
8. These signs are extremely complex and guides to them are readily available. See esp. the publications on *Umbanda* by Editôra Eco, Rio de Janeiro.
9. See Waite 1911:286. The authorship of this grimoire is obscure—see Summers 1945:133; Butler 1949:89. It is attributed to Pope Honorius III (1216–27).
10. Anon. (2) 18th cent.:99–100.
11. See above, page 27.
12. The *caboclo* Ogun can manifest himself under the name Ogun de lei, which according to Carneiro (1936:92) may be 'simples aférese de "Ogun de mâle" ...' *Pemba de lei* may have derived in like manner from *pemba de mâle*. The post-fix *de lei*, as transcribed above, also has

the sense of hallmarked or of acceptable quality as in *prata de lei* (hallmarked silver).

13. cf. Binon Cossard 1970:168–9, 253.
14. On one occasion C.4 remarked: 'I may well teach everything about *Candomblé*, but not prayers.'
15. cf. Rodrigues (1935:90). 'Isabel showed me some powders that had been made by her, which, when worn in amulets around the neck or even carried in the pocket, were sufficient to guarantee absolute happiness.'
16. For the *pade de Exú*, see above, page 32 n. 5. Street sellers of *acarajé* (fried maize cake) always make three small *acarajés* for Exú before cooking the rest. cf. Lima 1946:27.
17. *mangangá*: from the Tupi *mang-ã-caba* (wasp of high flight with a sting that produces fever).
18. A comparison may be drawn here between the dung beetle that comes under the control of Exú who brought fire and the sun (see above, page 38), and the Egyptian scarab beetle, which lays its egg in dung and then rolls it into a ball and pushes it into the sun. The ancient Egyptians associated this beetle with the god of creation and its egg-ball with the sun. The sun-god was called 'Roller' because he rolled the sun across the sky. See Wallis Budge 1930:135–6.
19. A large black bird that feeds on carrion: *Cathartes foetens*, C. (C.A.).
20. Type unknown. A powder to do evil made from a lizard is mentioned by Vasconcellos (1960:II, 105–6), who quotes the following variants from the *Romanceiro*, XL: *Veneno de Moriana* (Nos. 535 and 538 respectively):

    – Que fizeste ao teu vinho—que me fez tanto mal?
    – Deitei-lhe cobrinhas novas—pós de lagarto real.
    – Qu'é que lhe deitaste ò vinho—que me fez tanto mal?
    – Botei-lhe sangue de víbora—pó de lagarto moído.

21. cf. Querino 1938:88. See also João do Rio 1906:31—a pepper attached with black thread to a piece of paper bearing the name of the person involved and thrown into the fire will break that person's marriage.
22. The actual nest plays an important role in sorcery in that it is common for the sorcerer to place a piece of the intended victim's clothing inside a termite's nest, for example, and expect his victim to deteriorate at the same time as the cloth.

23. Barroso 1923:284–5 makes a comparison with the Japanese word for dragonfly. He quotes Lafcadio Hearn, *Kottô*, French translation by Joseph de Smet, Ed. Mercure de France, Paris 1912:182: 'Les libellules sont les chevaux des morts.'
24. Taboada 1947:46 and 1959:297; Amades 1951:111; Hildburgh 1951:244; but see esp. Thomas 1971:446, 517, 524, 547.
25. Pardal 1937:94. For the use of the toad in sorcery in Brazil, see Cabral 1942:268–9; Querino 1938:87.
26. For incantations to Exú, see Verger 1957:126–40.
27. A corruption of *Fierabras* (*Chanson de Geste* of the Charlemagne cycle—late twelfth, early thirteenth centuries). Fierabras is a giant and the son of the Saracen king, Balant. His name is associated with all that is powerful. Don Quijote, for example (Part I, Ch. XVII), is fortified with 'el bálsamo de Fierabrás y . . . con aquel remedio podía acometer desde allí adelante, sin temor alguno, cualesquiera ruinas, batallas y pendencias, por peligrosas que fuesen'. For the Portuguese, Ferrabraz has been almost synonymous with *mouro*: see Barroso (1949:31), who transcribes *Auto dos Fandangos* dating from the eighteenth century in which one of the characters is Ferrabraz, ambassador from Mauritania. In Brazil, Farrabás or Ferrabraz has subsequently become a synonym for Satan.
28. Beelzebub.
29. Maria Padrilha is one of the names given to Exú outside traditional *Candomblé*.
30. This is probably derived from traditional African belief that Exu's kingdom has either seven, fourteen or twenty-one roads crossing it. (See Bastide 1961:223.) In *Candomblé de caboclo*, this may have been transmogrified into a belief that there are twenty-one different Exús controlling these roads. The recipe given by C.6 (see Recipe E, pages 68–69, above) contains twenty-one ingredients.

CHAPTER IX. AMULETS

1. cf. Gardner 1942:102.
2. An amulet carved in the shape of a clenched fist with the thumb clasped between the fore and middle fingers.
3. cf. Wallis Budge 1930:29.
4. cf. Hardie (1923:163): '. . . their main purpose is apparently to divert to themselves the attention of any possible overlooker . . . The

amulets, in short, are a species of lightning conductor, just as the power of overlooking is thought popularly to be a kind of electricity which resides in the eye.'

5. Pires de Lima, quoted by Câmara Cascudo 1951:72. cf. Gardner 1942:97; Maclagan 1902 1st edn 1972:42; Hildburgh 1908:217–18, 1951:244–5.
6. See Vasconcellos 1892:8, 1925:28, 61, 65; Wallis Budge 1930: 316–17.
7. Transcribed in OSMA 1916:162. cf. Castillo de Lucas 1958:56.
8. cf. Hornell (1924:272), who mentions the custom in Trinidad of hanging jet beads around a child's wrist. If one of the beads breaks at any time, it is believed that the evil influence has passed into the bead. See also Vasconcellos 1925:65. Gifford (1958:78) quotes Gutiérrez, a Spanish physician, who in 1653 described a jet cross worn by his son to absorb malignant forces and which ultimately split.
9. OSMA *ibid.*
10. The fourth edition of the *Diccionário de Autoridades de la Lengua Castellana* (1803) describes *higa* as 'la mano derecha cortada al topo'; quoted by OSMA 1916:27, which gives illustrations of right-handed *figas* (pp. 21, 23). An illustration of a right-handed *figa* from Egypt is given by Wallis Budge 1930:172. See also Hansmann and Kriss-Rettenbeck 1966:199.
11. cf. Vasconcellos (1925:66), who mentions a similar practice in Portugal in order to attract custom.
12. Vianna Filho 1946:120; Lima 1946:88; Hoehne 1939:112–13.
13. Correa (1969:I, 180) and Câmara Cascudo (1951:71) mention the use of *arruda* for the manufacture of *figas* in Brazil. See also Bastide (1961:165) and Cunha (1941:42), who both mention the use of *guiné* for the manufacture of amulets. Maynard Araújo (1961:72–3) mentions that the most powerful form of *figa* is that made of *guiné* on a Friday. Costa (1907:108) says that *tipim* (*guiné*) is the best material for *figas*.
14. See particularly *Othello*, I, iii: 'Virtue! a fig! 'tis in ourselves that we are thus or thus.' And *Henry IV*, *Part Two*, V, iii: 'When Pistol lies, do this; and fig me, like the bragging Spaniard.'
15. Vasconcellos 1925:42–57.
16. Vasconcellos 1925:81–3.
17. Welsford 1968:61.
18. In Bahia, the plants *avenca* and *macaça* are believed to wilt if a

victim of the evil eye goes near them or even looks at them (C.1, C.5, S.6). cf. Hildburgh 1942:187.

19. This point has been stressed by numerous writers. See particularly Câmara Cascudo 1951:72; Vasconcellos 1925:20, 57–8; Maclagan 1902 1st edn 1972:4, 43; Hardie 1923:161; Freyre 1946:143. Note also Isaiah XIII: 18: 'their eye shall not spare children'.
20. This is the case during initiation rites when the neophyte is seen to be particularly exposed to danger on account of the fundamental change taking place in his or her status. Hence the complex rituals that must be performed. The blacksmith and the alchemist, as Eliade (1962:31, 102, 151) has pointed out, complete the process of creation by changing the status of metals and ores, but before commencing work they should undertake a whole series of rituals which will guarantee success. Maclagan (1902 1st edn 1972:72, 73, 78) gives three instances of failure to produce good butter when churning on account of the restricting forces of an evil eye.
21. cf. Cabral 1942:266; Taboada 1959:299; Risco 1961:82. Borrow (1841:I, 146) mentions the custom in Spain of children wearing a small horn tipped with silver.
22. See esp. Câmara Cascudo 1951:72; Silva 1926:11; Gouveia 1926: 47:8.
23. Hildburgh 1908:217–18.
24. cf. Vasconcellos 1892:9 and 1925:39.
25. See Rolleston 1943:292–3; Vasconcellos 1925:92.
26. For explanations of the system of divination with cowrie shells, see Bastide 1961:139ff.; Carneiro 1961:149–50; Frobenius 1973:183–91. For use of cowrie shells in Brazil in general, see Câmara Cascudo 1962:I, 146–7. Cult priests are able to distinguish between African and Brazilian cowrie shells, the former being considered much superior (C.5).
27. See Hildburgh 1942:178–9.
28. See Wallis Budge 1930:91, 141–2.
29. Maclagan 1902 1st edn 1972:19, 98–100; Castillo de Lucas 1958:56; Gifford 1958:65–6.
30. A similar distinction, for the same reasons, is made with onions.
31. Vasconcellos (1925:22) mentions the custom in Portugal of carrying garlic in the pocket to protect against the evil eye.
32. For possible origins of the pentangle, see Wallis Budge 1930:40, 233; Bouisson 1960:140–41.

33. cf. Vasconcellos 1892:5; Querino 1938:118–19; Ramos 1940:83.
34. See also Andrade 1963:136; Maynard Araújo 1958:88. I have also seen it painted on fishing boats in Galicia and north Portugal.
35. See below, Chapter XI, esp. pages 120–21. cf. Andrade (1963:122), who mentions drawing a pentangle on the floor at the start of a ritual to break up a love affair. There is a vast literature on the Cabbal. Spence (1921) summarizes the principal points.
36. cf. Waite (1911:101), who, quoting from the *Grand Grimoire*, mentions how Solomon forced all spirits to obey him by the power of his talisman. The Gnostics believed Solomon's seal worked miracles. See Wallis Budge 1930:203.
37. The number 5 is endowed with special qualities. For number symbolism in general, see Hopper 1938; Butler 1970.
38. cf. Teixeira 1954:33.
39. *ibid.* p. 22. See also Magalhães (1966:205–6), who quotes Pedro Sampaio's *A Medicina no Ceará*, p. 367; and Maynard Araújo 1958: 140.
40. See Querino 1938:118–19; Ramos 1940:83.
41. For the ring amulet, see Wallis Budge 1930:291–305.
42. cf. Vasconcellos 1892:8.
43. This is by no means certain, however, and it is stressed that the foregoing was only a theory put forward by certain Brazilian doctors. *Curandeiros* saw no link between *maniconia* and syphilis.
44. cf. Cabral 1942:266.
45. For information on herbs carried as amulets by South American Indians, see Safford 1917, esp. p. 424.
46. Câmara Cascudo 1962:II, 578–9.
47. Câmara Cascudo 1962:I, 135–6.
48. cf. Cabral 1942:267, 1957:170; Vasconcellos 1892:10.
49. See Pardal (1937:80), who quotes Catlin on the 'medicine bag': '. . . a la cual rinden el más grande homenaje y miran como la salvaguardia de su seguridad durante toda la vida . . . consideran que sin la bolsa, la mala suerte y las desdichas los acompañarán'.
50. According to legend, the Brazilian bandit Lampeão died because he had rendered his *patuá* powerless by wearing it when he was *de corpo sujo*. See Amorim 1959:225–6. cf. Campos 1967:31; Parrinder 1969: 159; Black 1883:170–71.
51. Talbot 1926:II, 180.
52. Parrinder 1969:160.

53. 'Os adultos porém, traziam pendentes do pescoço um patuá ou amulêto, pequena bolsa de couro contendo um objeto pertencente ao anjo da guarda . . .'
54. cf. Risco (1961:83), who describes an amulet consisting of the beginning of the four gospels enclosed in a silk bag and worn round the neck.
55. Alleged details concerning publication are: Rome, 1502 or 1522 (Gifford 1964:213). See also Waite 1911:41, 43.
56. Ramos 1940:83: '. . . não se separaram de seus talismans ou *mandingas*, e eram tidos como grandes feiticeiros, de onde o nome de *mandingueiros* por que se tornaram conhecidos'. See also Rodrigues 1935: 32; Querino 1938:118–19; Bouisson 1960:282.
57. Béart 1960:39; Parrinder 1969:161.
58. There is one Malé *seita* in Cachoeira which meets very rarely during the year. When the current *pai de santo* (C.10) dies, it will cease to function completely because there is no adequate successor.
59. cf. Maynard Araújo 1961:75.
60. Also given by Costa 1907:132.
61. Roughly equivalent to 'so-and-so'.
62. cf. the *curandeiro*'s use of water in a *sacudida;* see above, page 35.
63. This prayer is also quoted almost verbatim by Andrade 1963:210; Maynard Araújo 1958:132; Vieira Filho 1953–4:42.
64. For other prayers of this type, see Piazza 1960:123–4; Lima 1946:122, 123–4; Teixeira 1954:85; Boiteux 1944:41, 43. On p. 40, Boiteux gives a similar prayer with the words so arranged on the paper that they take the form of a cross. See also Cabral 1957:170.

Chapter X. The Reza (Curing Prayer)

1. cf. Rozeira (1963:556), who points out that a prayer to Santo Antonio de Lisboa is infallible when recited without any mistakes, but valueless when recited with errors.
2. Italics as in the original.
3. The *curandeiro*, however, tends to play both parts.
4. For similar versions, see Costa 1907:128; Lira 1944:281. For virtually identical versions which mention Sofia instead of Iria, see Gonçalves 1938:51; Magalhães 1966:219; and Vieira Filho 1953–4: 45. See also Braun 1950:57.
5. For a similar version, see Amorim 1959:137.

6. cf. Puckett (1926:368–9), who refers to a complaint known as 'fallen palate', cured by pulling the patient's hair sharply and striking the back of his neck.
7. See also Rodrigues 1907:274; Gouveia 1926:32; Cabral 1957:103; Lis Quibén 1949:497; Puckett 1926:374.
8. cf. Costa 1907:128–9; Magalhães 1966:198–9; Oliveira 1948:85–6; Cunha 1951:9; Cabral 1957:104.
9. See Maynard Araújo 1958:137; Teixeira 1954:36–8.
10. The two saints may have identical or very similar names, e.g.:

    'Santa Iria perguntou a Santa Iria
    Cobreiro bravo com que se curaria.
    Com ramo verde e agua fria,
    Com o nome de Deus e da Virgem Maria,
    Só com isso se curaria.' [Nunes 1950:44]

    'São Andrão perguntou a Santa Andria
    Cobreiro brabo com que se curaria
    — Com ramo verde e agua fria
    Em nome de Deus e da Virgem Maria.' [Paula 1951:27]

    'Santo Egídio perguntô pra Santa Egida:—Com que se cura impige ou cobrêro? Arrespondeu Santa Egida:—Com funcho e água fria, Padre Nosso e Ave-Maria.' (Teixeira 1954:38).
11. Examples of such types may be found in Boiteux 1944:35, 36; Campos 1967:118; Gouveia 1926:33, 34; Magalhães 1966:200–201; Romero 1954:673. For other curing prayers using different techniques, see Paz 1954:75, 76; Braun 1950:57; Campos 1967:119; Nunes 1950:43, 44, 47; Valle 1963:607–8.
12. Probably a corruption of *enxaqueca* = migraine.
13. Described by S.1 as a sudden sharp pain.
14. For other prayers for headaches but which bear no resemblance to the one transcribed, see Amorim 1959:139; Maynard Araújo 1961:340–41; Lima 1946:117–18.
15. Saint Apollonia.
16. For variations, see Amorim 1959:142–3; Boiteux 1944:35; Campos 1967:130; César 1941:153: Lima 1946:119–20; Teixeira 1954:44; Vieira Filho 1953–4:46. For other prayers for toothache, see Barroso 1949:441; Cabral 1957:141–4; Gomes 1951:191; Gouveia 1926: 86; Vasconcellos 1882:20; Magalhães 1966:228; Nunes 1950:45; Paula 1951:29; Silva 1926:23.

17. cf. Piazza (1960:129), who gives a prayer for toothache addressed to the waxing moon. cf. also Cabral (1957:142), who records the general belief that toothache could derive from prolonged exposure to the sun.
18. cf. the versions of this legend and examples of prayers given by Campos 1967:120–21; Amorim 1959:135–6; Magalhães 1966:208; Teixeira 1954:49; Paz 1954:73. Other sources quote variations on the above in which São Braz (or Brás) is also asked to intercede, e.g.: 'São Brás Bispo/Homem bom e mulher má/Esteira velha e ceia má/Foi Deus Nosso Senhor quem disse/Que és de desengasgar' (Gonçalves 1938:51). For other examples of this, see Amorim 1959:137; Campos 1967:121; César 1941:166; Nunes 1950:44; Romero 1954: II, 671.
19. For variations, see Cabral 1957:124; Gouveia 1926:27; Amorim 1959:135; Birnfeld 1951:59; Magalhães 1966:208.
20. cf. Dietschy (1939:20), who mentions that the Incas used to use llama wool and feathers in order to arrest bleeding. Braun (1950:56–7) mentions using a chicken feather. Paula (1951:28) records the use of lamb's wool. Black wool and butter were prescribed in Britain 'probably for unction' (Black 1883:117). See also Lis Quibén 1945: 275, 276, 285.
21. cf. Lis Quibén 1945:285–6, 1949:310–11; Carneiro e Lima 1943:16, 26ff.
22. cf. Cabral 1957:95.
23. Magalhães (1966:222) quotes Rodrigues, who mentions how keeping a *jaboti* turtle in the house helps to cure *erisipela*. He suggests this may be indigenous in origin. cf. Lima (1946:92): 'Ter um cágado em casa evita a entrada dos malefícios.'
24. Similar versions, sometimes involving different saints on a different journey, are given by Campos 1967:127–9; Dias 1944:I, 169–70; Gonçalves 1938:40; Vasconcellos 1906:III, 196; Paula 1951:28; Lis Quibén 1945:274–6, 278, 714; Maynard Araújo 1958:138; Teixeira 1954:51, 53–4; Valle 1963:600–602; Carneiro e Lima 1943: 16ff.
25. Similar versions are given by Teixeira 1954:53; Nunes 1950:47; Magalhães 1966:223; Campos 1960:132, Boiteux 1944:37; Barroso 1949:444.
26. For other definitions of *espinhela caída*, see esp. Piso 1648:22–3; Campos 1967:56–7; Magalhães 1966:225; Gonçalves 1938:39; São Paulo 1970:I, 141–7.

27. Amorim (1959:139) records an identical method. Lis Quibén (1945: 288, 293, 714) compares the measurements of each of the patient's hands, arms and legs. Rodríguez López (1974:119–20) compares the lengths of the patient's arms.
28. For similar versions, see Campos 1967:112–13; César 1941:159; Edmundo 1932:474; Magalhães 1966:226; Paula 1952:17.
29. cf. Boiteux 1944:36–7.
30. cf. Lima 1946:128; Teixeira 1954:55.
31. Maynard Araújo (1958:65) uses the term to describe diarrhoea. cf. Vogel (1970:188–9), who mentions how the terms 'flux' or 'bloody flux' were applied to dysentery in North America. See also Cabral 1957:128.
32. The sense here is unclear, and the translation attempts only an approximation of the true meaning.
33. For variations, see Amorim 1959:139–40; Boiteux 1944:35, 41; Campos 1967:125; César 1941:149; Costa 1907:127–9; Gonçalves 1938:37; Gouveia 1926:86; Lima 1946:118; Magalhães 1966:203–4; Paula 1952:16; Piazza 1960:121. A very similar prayer in Latin is given by McKenzie 1927:74.
34. For variations, see Barroso 1949:441; Boiteux 1944:37; Braun 1950: 57; Campos 1967:132; Costa 1907:18–19; Magalhães 1966:205; Nunes 1950:44; Valle 1963:603.
35. For variations, see Campos 1967:131; Magalhães 1966: 206–7.
36. Vieira Filho (1953–4:46) gives a prayer that cures either erysipelas or the evil eye.
37. cf. Maynard Araújo 1961:64–5 (*arruda* or *guiné*); Cabral 1957:176 (*arruda* or *alecrim*), 1942:226 (*arruda*). Teixeira (1954:89) mentions one instance when *Maria preta* should be used for a boy, *mentraço* (*mentrasto*) for a girl. However, *arruda* may be used for both sexes. Vieira Filho 1953–4:45 (*arruda*).
38. For a similar comparison, see Vasconcellos 1882:101. Vieira Filho (1953–4:46) gives the variation, 'Tu és ferro, eu sou osso.' Campos (1967:122–3) gives a further variation: 'Tu és a madeira e eu sou o machado, tu és a fera e eu sou a espada.'
39. 'Two' refers to the two eyes, and 'three' to the three sprigs of herbs held by the reciter.
40. The spirit of a dead person who haunts the living. See below, page 108.
41. *encorrentar*: in spirit sessions, when all the mediums are possessed

they join hands and invite the sick people present to join hands with them. It is believed that a current emanating from the mediums will pass through the sick people and cleanse them. The word *encorrentar* is used to describe this.

42. A medium is believed when possessed to have the power spiritually to cleanse others who are present. The person concerned stands in front of the medium, exchanges a few words of greeting with the spirit possessing the medium and sometimes asks advice. Then the medium spins him round three times to the left and three times to the right, hits the soles of each foot three times, pulls each finger until the joint cracks and finally blows in each ear. The ritual is known as *passe*.
43. For other prayers for the evil eye, see Campos 1967:122–4; Vieira Filho 1953–4:46; Lima 1946:88–9; Maynard Araújo 1961:65–6; Nunes 1950:46; Orico 1937:208; Paula 1952:18; Piazza 1960:122; Teixeira 1954:88–92; Dias 1944:I, 168–9; Lis Quibén 1945:258, 310–11; Valle 1963:598.
44. For variations, see Braun 1950:58–9; Cabral 1957:110; Magalhães 1966:232; Maynard Araújo 1958:140; Lira 1944:281; Teixeira 1954:97.
45. For variations, see Boiteux 1944:35–6; Cabral 1957:111–12; Campos 1967:132; Costa 1907:128; Vieira Filho 1953–4:45; Gomes 1951:191; Gouveia 1926:26; Vasconcellos 1906:III, 203; Magalhães 1966:230, 232.
46. For variations, see Maynard Araújo 1958:140. Lis Quibén (1945:694–6, 704) mentions Santa Lucia's three needles, the third of which she uses to take specks of dust out of the eye.
47. cf. Nunes 1950:44.
48. For variations, see Gonçalves 1938:36; Magalhães 1966:212; Campos 1967:131; Maynard Araújo 1961:217.
49. This prayer may also be worn in a *patuá* during pregnancy.
50. For variations, see Boiteux 1944:36; Paula 1951:28. Teixeira (1954:102–3) gives a version that mentions Santa Aurora instead of Santa Sofia.
51. cf. Valle (1963:611), who says that in Gulpilhares (Portugal) it should only be done between 11 and 12 a.m.; and Paula (1951:29), who says it should never be done in the morning or at midday, but only after 3 p.m.
52. For variations of the above prayers, see Birnfeld 1951:60; Boiteux

1944:36; Cabral 1957:150; Campos 1967:116–18; César 1941:151; Paula 1951:29; Teixeira 1954:27. Other prayers for *sol na cabeça* are given by Braun 1950:57; Gouveia 1926:80–81; Teixeira 1954:26; Valle 1963:611; Vieira Filho 1953–4:44.

53. For variations, see Braun 1950:57; Nunes 1950:46.
54. cf. Cabral 1957:159; Birnfeld 1951:59–60; Braun 1950:59; Campos 1967:113–14.
55. For variations, see Barroso 1949:443; Boiteux 1944:35; Braun 1950:59; Cabral 1957:159; Campos 1967:113–15; César 1941:164; Lima 1946:118; Magalhães 1966:237; Nunes 1950:45; Paula 1951:29; Teixeira 1954:115–19; Valle 1963:603.
56. cf. Lis Quibén 1949:310.
57. cf. Lis Quibén 1949:475–9.
58. See also Cunha 1951:9; Maynard Araújo 1961:54–5; Teixeira 1954:130; Cabral 1957:146.
59. The idea that an ill wind brings misfortunes is common to many cultures. Pardal (1937:156–7) points out how, in Quechua, words for certain illnesses are based on the word for 'air' (*huaira*). Hence *aya-huaira* (epilepsy), *cceho-huaira* (tetanus), etc. See also Magalhães 1966:25 in this connection. Similarly, among the Nahua (Mexico) there is a sickness known as *aire* or *aigre* which strikes when certain spirits known as *enanitos* or *aires* blow their breath on humans (Madsen 1969:629).
60. I was unable to ascertain why this should be so. (S.1) suggested that it was out of respect for the day in the week on which Christ died.
61. 'Caw' is translated literally from the Portuguese *gorgoveia*, which is a corruption of *corveja*. The verb here should in fact be *balir* (to bleat). See also below, page 111.
62. For other prayers against the *vento mal*, see Vasconcellos 1882:52–3; Boiteux 1944:42; Magalhães 1966:35–6; Maynard Araújo 1958:137–8; Lis Quibén 1949:474.
63. Maynard Araújo (1961:221) mentions how mothers are constantly on the watch for symptoms of *ventre caído* in their children.
64. cf. Lis Quibén 1949:331–2.
65. cf. Teixeira 1954:120.
66. For other prayers, see Amorim 1959:137; Campos 1967:122; Lis Quibén 1945:323; Taboada 1947:44; Teixeira 1954:120–22.
67. cf. Piazza 1949:17; Taboada 1947:45; 1949:113.
68. cf. Cabral 1957:114; Magalhães 1966:217. For other prayers for

warts, see Boiteux 1944:39; Braun 1950:57; Campos 1967:131–2; Paula 1952:17; Lis Quibén 1949:505–6.

69. cf. Campos (1967:117–18), who quotes Mário Ypiranga Monteiro (no details) as saying that references to the *mar sagrado* in prayers are 'puro candomblé'. This is doubtful, since the expression does appear in curing prayers in Portugal.
70. cf. Carneiro and Pires de Lima 1943:17: 'Na linguagem familiar, a frase *seja Pedro ou Paulo* significa "seja quem for".' (In everyday speech the phrase 'be it Peter or Paul' means 'whoever it may be').
71. See above, pages 27 and 29–30.

Chapter XI. Ebó

1. See esp. Bastide 1961:355; Querino 1955:78–9.
2. cf. Carneiro 1936:132.
3. Balls of ground maize cooked in water and wrapped in banana leaves. Lima (1946:44), quoting Sodré Viana *Caderno de Xangô* (no details), gives the following recipe: 'Put any quantity of maize stripped from the cob—the white or red variety—in cold water to soften it. When it is swollen, grind it at the finest setting. Season the dough with a little salt and put it in a pan with water to cook. Wrap small quantities —not much more than a medium-size cupful—in green banana leaves and let it cool. Serve wrapped in the little parcels of leaves.' *Acaçá* can be red or white, depending on the type of maize used.
4. See St Clair 1971:127ff., and his photographs facing *ibid.*:160.
5. See Verger 1957:88–9; Querino 1955:76–7.
6. People possessed for the first time are often flung to the ground by the *orixá*, hence *queda* (fall).
7. Bastide's article (1950) should be consulted for more details concerning the cure of illness that originates in neglect of ritual or failure on the part of the patient to seek initiation into the cult.
8. The medium is not at all aware of what words were spoken when he or she was possessed.
9. The average exchange rate when these figures were supplied (1973–4) was £1.00 = Cr $15.00.
10. Before the start of an *egun* cult festival on the island of Itaparica, it is common for one of the priests to leave a tray on the floor in front of the onlookers. Those who later in the evening are going to consult the *egun* spirits, place an offering on the tray. Sometimes the tray is

flung into the room (where the festival is to take place) through the space under a closed door, it being believed by all present that the tray was flung by an *egun*. Such funds, also called *dinheiro do chão*, go towards the upkeep of the cult house and the elaborate costumes worn by the *egun* (I.4, I.5).

11. See Appendix Four.
12. Ogun's sword hilt is always as follows:

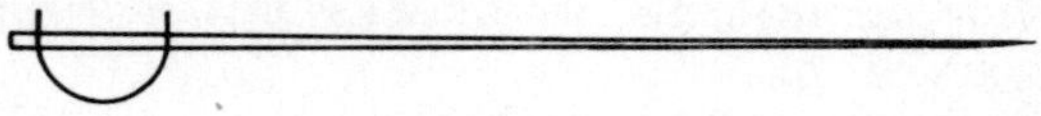

Ogun and Yansan are easily distinguished in this way.

13. The soul or spirit in the form of a bird is a common symbol in many religions: 'Often the soul is conceived as a bird ready to take flight. This conception has probably left traces in most languages, and it lingers as a metaphor in poetry. The Malays carry out the conception of the bird-soul in a number of odd ways. If the soul is a bird on the wing, it may be attracted by rice, and so either prevented from flying away or lured back again from its perilous flight. Thus in Java when a child is placed on the ground for the first time (a moment which uncultured people seem to regard as especially dangerous), it is put in a hencoop and the mother makes a clucking sound, as if she were calling hens. And in Sintang, a district of Borneo, when a person, whether man, woman, or child, has fallen out of a house or off a tree, and has been brought home, his wife or other kinswoman goes as speedily as possible to the spot where the accident happened, and there strews rice, which has been coloured yellow, while she utters the words "Cluck! cluck! soul! So-and-so is in his house again. Cluck! cluck! soul!" Then she gathers up the rice in a basket, carries it to the sufferer, and drops the grains from her hand on his head, saying again, "Cluck! cluck! soul!" Here the intention is clearly to decoy back the loitering bird-soul and replace it in the head of its owner' (Frazer 1922 1st edn 1971:239).
14. Again, in this instance, *discarrego* should read *descarregamento*, meaning unburdening.
15. Confusion such as this between the *egun* and Exú is very typical in *Candomblé de caboclo*, but never found in the traditional *seitas*.
16. *Pemba* here refers to *pemba preta*, assumed by the *mãe* to be the cause of the patient's illness.
17. The cry of salutation of Exú.
18. These numbers may be interchanged.

19. Another *caboclo* spirit. See above, page 18.
20. The *pai* here is requesting the additional power of the stars, water and the jungle to assist him in bringing about a cure. This particular informant (C.2) conducted further rituals after the *trabalho* embodying these three additional elements. This is described below, pages 130–33.
21. Another title for Ogun.
22. Boiadeiro, Jurema and Sultão das Matas are *caboclo* spirits. See above, page 18.
23. *Babalorixá : pai de santo.*
24. Cry of salutation for Abaluayé.
25. Babá (Yoruba): father.
26. An affectionate term of address for Abaluayé.
27. An example of how a traditional African *orixá* can be fused with a *caboclo* spirit, calling itself 'Obaluayé de caboclo'.
28. Despite references to cutting in this prayer, the cotton is not actually cut by the *pai* until towards the end of the *trabalho*. See below, page 129.
29. Another title for Naná. See Verger 1957:274, 280–81.
30. Another *caboclo* spirit, See above, page 18.
31. 'Village' (Port. *aldeia*) is also used to designate a cult house.
32. Cry of salutation for Xangô. Xangô and Yansan (Saint Barbara) are closely linked in their functions as *orixás*, hence Xangô is mentioned in this manner at the end of an incantation dedicated to Saint Barbara.
33. Obaluayé may be substituted by Senhor Oxossi or Ogun.
34. In other spirit sessions, however, when the primary objective was not to cure, I sometimes witnessed mediums possessed by the spirits of recently dead local people, though this type of spirit was certainly in the minority. In the majority of cases, most spirits were familiar *orixás* or *caboclos*.
35. A form of *pade de Exú* designed to ward off evil forces until the end of the ceremony.
36. i.e. the candles.
37. Another title for Oxossi (C.2's *orixá*).
38. If the ceremony takes place on a beach by the sea, the food is that of Yemanjá; if on the banks of a river, it is that of Oxun. In Cachoeira, where this ceremony was witnessed, the river is tidal, so both goddesses are invoked.

Conclusion

1. For more information on Arigó and Doctor Fritz, see St Clair 1971: 116ff.

Appendix Four. The Question of Payment

1. Various sources support this view, Cf. Lima 1946:14; Maynard Araújo 1958:148; 1961:93, 99, 145, 191; Oliveira 1948:87; Pierson 1951:149.

Appendix Six. Personal Details Concerning Informants

1. Numerous divisions and sub-divisions of colour are made in Brazil for official and non-official purposes. Wagley (1963) discusses these and their implications in detail. For the purposes of this study it is considered sufficient to use four groupings: black, dark *mulato*, light *mulato* and white.
2. God, i.e. the god to whom a person may be dedicated within the terms of the *Candomblé* religion. This point has been discussed in full (see pp. 13ff.).
3. Divorce as such is not permitted in Brazil, but legal separation, *desquite*, is recognized and provisions are made under the law for *desquitados*.
4. *Mãe de santo* = a high priestess in the *Candomblé* cult. Similarly, *pai de santo* = a high priest. Literally the terms mean mother of the saints and father of the saints, saints here referring to African deities. This is discussed on page 14.
5. Cult house.
6. *Mãe pequena*: assistant to the *mãe de santo*.
7. This case is an exception in that the woman had no black blood. *Mulata* here refers purely to her colour.
8. *Filha de santo*: initiated and fully participant female cult member. Literally 'daughter of the saints'.
9. *Ogã*: holder of post of responsibility within the *terreiro*.
10. Again, the term *mulato* here can only indicate colour and not ethnic origin as this informant was of pure Indian extraction.

BIBLIOGRAPHY

Abbreviations used in bibliography and in notes and references

A.A.: American Anthropologist
A.C.: Actas Ciba (n.p.; São Paulo?)
A.C.I.E.: Actas do Congresso Internacional de Etnografia—promovido pela Câmara Municipal de Santo Tirso de 10 a 18 de julho de 1963
C.A.: Dicionário Caldas Aulete
C.L.A.L.S.: Centre for Latin American Linguistic Studies, University of St Andrews
H.S.A.I.: Handbook of South American Indians (Washington)
I.B.G.E.: Instituto Brasileiro de Geografia e Estatística
J.A.F.: Journal of American Folklore
J.A.S.: Journal of Asian Studies
J.R.A.I.: Journal of the Royal Anthropological Institute
n.d.: no date of publication given
n.p.: no place of publication given
O.E.D.: Oxford English Dictionary
R.A.M.: Revista do Arquivo Municipal (São Paulo)
R.D.T.P.: Revista de Dialectologia y Tradiciones Populares
R.E.: Revista de Etnografia (Porto)
R.I.H.G.B.: Revista do Instituto Histórico e Geográfico Brasileiro
S.C.C.F.: Sub-Comissão Catarinense de Folclore: Boletim Trimestral

Alvarez Bláquez, Darío, Dr, 'Algunos Aciertos de la Medicina Popular Galaico-Portuguesa', in *A.C.I.E.*, 13–22.
Amades, J., Piedras de Virtud, *R.D.T.P.*, Vol. VII, 1951, 84–131.
Amorim, José Pimentel de, 'Medicina Popular em Alagoas', *R.A.M.*, Vol. CLXII, 1959, 129–240.
Andrade, Luiz de, 'Raizes Psicológicas dos Cultos do Fogo', *R.A.M.*, Vol. CLXII, 1959, 241–93.
Andrade, Mario de, *Música de Feitiçaria no Brasil*, São Paulo, 1963.
Anon. (1), *La Véritable Magie Noire ou le Secret des Secrets*, Rome, 1750.
Anon. (2), *Le Grand Grimoire, avec la Grande Clavicule de Salomon, Et la Magie Noire, ou les forces infernales du Grand Agrippa, pour découvrir tous les trésors cachés, et se faire obéir par tous les Esprits; suivie de tous les Arts Magiques*, n.p., n.d. (18th cent.?).
Azevedo, Fernando de, *A Cultura Brasileira—Introdução ao estudo da Cultura no Brasil*, São Paulo, 1964.
Azevedo, Thales de, *Povoamento da Cidade do Salvador*, Salvador, 1969.
Barriola, Ignacio Maria, *La Medicina Popular en el País Vasco*, San Sebastián, 1952.
Barroso, Gustavo, *O Sertão e o Mundo*, Rio de Janeiro, 1923.

——, *Através dos Folk-lores*, São Paulo, 1927.
——, *Ao Som da Viola*, Rio da Janeiro, 1949.
Bascom, William R., 'The Focus of Cuban Santería', *South-Western Journal of Anthropology*, Vol. 6, 1950, 64–8.
Bastide, Roger, 'Medicina e Magia nos Candomblés', Separata de *Boletim Bibliográfico*, No. XVI, São Paulo, 1950.
——, *O Candomblé da Bahia* (*Rito Nagô*), São Paulo, 1961. Trans. by María Isaura Pereira de Queiroz. (Originally published, Mouton & Co., The Hague, 1958.)
——, *Les Religions africaines au Brésil*, Paris, 1960.
——, *Estudos Afro-Brasileiros*, São Paulo, 1973.
Béart, Charles, *Recherche des éléments d'une sociologie des peuples africains à partir de leurs jeux*, Paris, 1960.
Binon Cossard, Gisèle, *Contribution à l'étude des Candomblés au Brésil. Le Candomblé Angola*, Doctorat de Troisième Cycle (Directeur de Recherches: Roger Bastide). Unpublished thesis, 1970.
Birnfeld, Mário Campos, 'Tia Chica', *S.C.C.F.*, No. 8, 1951, 58–60.
Blache, Marta, 'El Curanderismo Folklórico enfocado a través de los procesos legales', in *A.C.I.E.*, 1963, 29–73.
Black, W. G., *Folk-Medicine*, London, 1883.
Boiteux, Lucas A., 'Poranduba Catarinense', *R.I.H.G.B.*, Vol. 184, Rio de Janeiro, 1944, 3–92.
Borges, T. Pompeu Accioly, *Migraçoes Internas no Brasil*, Rio de Janeiro, 1955.
Borrow, G., *The Zincali*, Vols. I–II, London, 1841.
Bouisson, Maurice, *Magic: Its Rites and History*, London, 1960. Trans. by G. Almayrac.
Bouza Brey, F., 'El Lagarto en la Tradición Popular Gallega', *R.D.T.P.*, Vol. V, 1949, 531–50.
Braun, Padre Alvino Bertholdo, 'Folclore e a Escola', *S.C.C.F.*, No. 5, 1950, 56–9.
Burton, Sir Richard Francis, *Explorations of the Highlands of Brazil*, Vols. I–II, London, 1869.
Burton, Robert, *Anatomy of Melancholy*, Oxford, 1628.
Butler, Christopher, *Number Symbolism*, London, 1970.
Butler, E. M., *Ritual Magic*, Cambridge, 1949.
Cabral, Oswaldo R., *Medicina, Medicos e Charlatães do Passado*, Florianópolis, 1942.
——, 'A Medicina Teológica e as Benzeduras', *R.A.M.*, Vol. CLX, 1957, 5–204.
Câmara Cascudo, Luís da, *Meleagro—depoimento e pesquisa sôbre a magia branca no Brasil*, Rio de Janeiro, 1951.
——, 'Promessa de Jantar aos Cães', *R.D.T.P.*, Vol. XIV, 1958, 14–17.
——, *Dicionário do Folclore Brasileiro*, Vols. I–II, Rio de Janeiro, 1962.
——, 'História da Alimentação no Brasil', *R.E.*, No. 1, Vol. 1, July 1963, 47–53.
——, *Made in Africa*, Rio de Janeiro, 1965.
Campos, Eduardo, *Folclore do Nordeste*, Rio de Janeiro, 1960.
——, *Medicina Popular do Nordeste*, Rio de Janeiro, 1967.

Cardinall, A. W., *The Natives of the Northeastern Territories of the Gold Coast*, London, n.d.
Cardoner Planas, A., 'Los Talismanes y la Patología Medieval', *R.D.T.P.*, Vol. XIV, 1958, 52–69.
Carneiro, Alexandre Lima, and Pires de Lima, Fernando de Castro, *Arte de Talher a Erisipela*, Porto, 1943.
Carneiro, Edison, *Religiões Negras*, Rio de Janeiro, 1936.
——, *Candomblés da Bahia*, Rio de Janeiro, 1961.
Carrington Bolton, Henry, *The Counting Out Rhymes of Children—Their Antiquity, Origin and Wide Distribution*, London, 1888.
Carus, P., *The History of the Devil and the Idea of Evil*, London, 1900.
Castillo de Lucas, Antonio, 'Terapeutica Ocular', *S.C.C.F.*, No. 8, 1951, 97–8.
——, *Folkmedicina*, Madrid, 1958.
——, 'Hagiografía Folklórico-Medica de San Juan Bautista', *R.E.*, No. 1, Vol. 2, Oct. 1963, 304–20.
César, Getulio, *Crendices do Nordeste*, São Paulo, 1941.
Clodd, Edward, *Magic in Names and in Other Things*, London, 1920.
Cointe, Paul le, *A Amazonia Brasileira—Arvores e Plantas Uteis*, Belém, 1934.
Correa, M. Pio, *Dicionário das Plantas Úteis do Brasil*, Rio de Janeiro, 1969. (Only Vols. I–IV [A–L] have so far been issued.)
Costa, Francisco Augusto Pereira da, 'Folk-lore Pernambucano', *R.I.H.G.B.*, Vol. LXX, part II, 1907, 7–641.
Culpeper, N., *The Complete Herbal*, London, 1850. (First published, 1653.)
Cunha, Narciso Soares da, *De von Martius aos Ervanários da Bahia*, Bahia, 1941.
Cunha, Rui Vieira da, 'Vocabulário de Consultório Médico', *S.C.C.F.*, No. 7, 1951, 8–9.
Curry, W. C., *Chaucer and the Mediaeval Sciences*, London, 1960.
Danzel, Th. W., *Magie et science secrète*, Paris, 1947.
Dawson, G. G., *Healing: Pagan and Christian*, London, 1935.
Debret, J. B., *Viagem Pitoresca e Histórica ao Brasil*, Vols. I and II, n.d., São Paulo.
Dias, Jaime Lopes, *Etnografía da Beira*, Vols. I–XI, Vol. I, Lisbon, 1944.
Dietschy, Hans, 'O Médico do Tempo dos Incas e Seus Remédios', *A.C.*, 4, 1939, 20.
Douglas, Mary, *Purity and Danger—An Analysis of Concepts of Pollution and Taboo*, London, 1970. (First published, London, 1966.)
——, *Natural Symbols—Explorations in Cosmology*, London, 1973. (First published, London, 1970.)
Edmundo, Luiz, *O Rio de Janeiro no Tempo dos Vice-Reis*, Rio de Janeiro, 1932.
Eduardo, Octavio da Costa, *The Negro in Northern Brazil*, Seattle and London, 1966.
Eliade, M., *The Forge and the Crucible*, London, 1962. Trans. from the French by S. Corrin. (First published, Paris, 1956.)
——, *Myths, Dreams and Mysteries: the Encounter Between Contemporary Faiths and Archaic Reality*, London, 1972. Trans. from the French by Philip Mairet. (First published Paris, 1957).
Elworthy, F. T., *The Evil Eye*, London, 1895.

Etienne, L'abbé Ignace, 'La Secte musulmane des Malès du Brésil et leur révolte en 1835', *Anthropos*, 1909, 99–105, 405–15.
Fernandes, Florestan, *A integração do negro à sociedade de classes*, São Paulo, 1964.
Findlay, J. A., *On the Edge of the Etheric*, London, 1931.
Ford, R., *A Handbook for Travellers in Spain*, Part I, London, 1845.
Frazer, J. G., *The Golden Bough: A Study in Magic and Religion*, London, 1971. (First published, London, 1922.)
Freyre, Gilberto, *The Masters and the Slaves*, New York, 1946. Trans. S. Putnam. (First published, Rio de Janeiro, 1933.)
——, *The Mansions and the Shanties*, New York, 1963. Trans. H. de Onís. (First published, Rio de Janeiro, 1936.)
Frobenius, Léo, *Léo Frobenius 1873–1973—An Anthology*, ed. Eike Haberland, Wiesbaden, 1973.
Gallet, Luciano, *Estudos de Folclore*, Rio de Janeiro, 1934.
Gardner, G., *Travels in the Interior of Brazil*, London, 1846.
Gardner, G. B., 'British Charms, Amulets and Talismans', *Folklore*, Vol. LIII, 1942, 95–103.
Gifford, D. J., 'An Early White Paternoster in Basque?', *Bulletin of Hispanic Studies*, Vol. XL1, 1964, 209–22.
Gifford, E. S., *The Evil Eye*, New York, 1958.
Gomes, Antonio Osmar, *Tradições Populares Colhidas no Baixo São Francisco*, Rio de Janeiro, 1951.
Gomes, Bernardino Antonio, *Plantas Medicinais do Brasil*, São Paulo, 1972. (First published, Rio de Janeiro, 1809.)
Gonçalves, Fernandes, *O Folklore Mágico do Nordeste—usos, costumes, crenças e ofícios mágicos das populações nordestinas*, Rio de Janeiro, 1938.
Gouveia, Daniel, *Folklore Brasileiro*, Rio de Janeiro, 1926.
Granada, Daniel, *Reseña histórico-descriptiva de antiguas y modernas supersticiones del Río de la Plata*, Montevideo, 1897.
Gubbins, J. K., 'Some Observations on the Evil Eye in Modern Greece', *Folklore*, Vol. LVII, 1946, 195–8.
Hansmann, L. and Kriss-Retenbeck, L., *Amulett und Talisman*, Munich, 1966.
Hardie, M. M., 'The Evil Eye in Some Greek Villages of the Upper Haliakmon Valley in West Macedonia', *J.R.A.I.*, Vol. LIII, 1923, 160–72.
Harper, E. B., 'Ritual Pollution as an Integrator of Caste and Religion', *J.A.S.*, Vol. 23, 1964, 151–97.
Henshall, J. D., and Momsen, R. P., *A Geography of Brazilian Development*, London, 1974.
Herskovits, M. J., 'African Gods and Catholic Saints in New World Negro Belief', *A.A.*, No. 39, 1937, 635–43.
——, 'Southernmost Outposts of New World Africanisms', *A.A.*, No. 45, 1943, 495–510.
——, 'Afroamerican Studies and Africanist Research', *A.A.*, No. 50, 1948, 1–10.
——, *The Myth of the Negro Past*. Boston, 1967.
Hildburgh, W. L., 'Notes on Spanish Amulets', *Folklore*, Vol. XVII, 1906, 454–71.

——, 'Notes on Some Contemporary Portuguese Amulets', *Folklore*, Vol. XIX, 1908, 213–24.

——, 'Further Notes on Spanish Amulets', *Folklore*, Vol. XXIV, 1913, 63–74.

——, 'Notes on Spanish Amulets (Third Series)', *Folklore*, Vol. XXV, 1914, 206–12.

——, 'Notes on Spanish Amulets (Fourth Series)', *Folklore*, Vol. XXVI, 1915, 404–16.

——, ' "Caravaca" Crosses and Their Uses as Amulets in Spain', *Folklore*, Vol. LI, 1940, 241–58.

——, 'Cowrie Shells as Amulets in Europe', *Folklore*, Vol. LIII, 1942, 178–95.

——, 'Psychology Underlying the Employment of Amulets in Europe', *Folklore*, Vol. LXII, 1951, 231–51.

——, 'Some Spanish Amulets Connected with Lactation', *Folklore*, Vol. LXII, 1951, 430–48.

Hoehne, F. C., *Botanica e Agricultura no Brasil no Seculo XVI*, São Paulo, 1937.

——, *Plantas e Substancias Vegetais Tóxicas e Medicinais*, São Paulo, 1939.

Hole, Christina, 'Superstitions and Beliefs of the Sea', *Folklore*, Vol. 78, 1967, 184–9.

Hopper, Vincent Foster, *Medieval Number Symbolism*, New York, 1938.

Hornell, J., 'The Evil Eye and Related Beliefs in Trinidad', *Folklore*, Vol. XXXV, 1924, 270–75.

Huizinga, J., *Homo Ludens*, São Paulo, 1971. Trans. João Paulo Monteiro. (First published, Switzerland, 1944.)

Hutchinson, Harry William, *Village and Plantation Life in Northeastern Brazil*, Seattle, 1957.

Izquierdo, Juliana, 'Oraciones de Pedroñeras (Cuenca)', *R.D.T.P.*, Vol. VI, 1950, 502–3.

João do Rio, Paulo Barreto, *As Religiões no Rio*, Rio de Janeiro, 1906.

Karsten, R., *The Civilization of the South American Indians*, London, 1926.

Koster, H., *Travels in Brazil 1809–1815*, Vols. I and II, London, 1816.

Krappe, A. H., *The Science of Folklore*, London, 1962. (First published, London, 1930.)

Léry, Jean de, *Histoire d'un voyage fait en la terre du Brésil*, Lausanne, 1972.

Lévi-Strauss, C., *The Raw and the Cooked*, London, 1970. (First published, Paris, 1964.)

——, *From Honey to Ashes*, London, 1973. (First published, Paris, 1966.)

Lévy-Bruhl, L., *How Natives Think*, London, 1926. Trans. L. Clare. (Original French edition entitled *Les Fonctions mentales dans les sociétés inférieures*.)

Lima, José, *Folk-lore Baiano (Tres ensaios)*, Bahia, 1946.

——, *A Festa de Egun e outros ensaios—resas, meisinhas, mandingas e mandingueiros da Bahia*, Rio de Janeiro, n.d.

Lima, Rossini Tavares de, 'A Malhação de Judas em São Paulo', *R.A.M.*, Vol. CLXIII, 1959, 9–38.

Lira, Jorge A., *Farmacopea Tradicional Indigena y Practicas Rituales*, Lima, 1946.

——, 'Diccionario Kkechuwa-Español', in *Revista del Museo Nacional*, Vol. XXIX, Lima, 1960, 29–47.

Lira, Marisa, 'Rezas e Feitiços', *Revista Filológica*, No. 27, 1944, 276–83.

——, *Estudos de Folclore Luso-Brasileiro*, Rio de Janeiro, 1952.

Lis Quibén, 'Medicina Popular Gallega', *R.D.T.P.*, No. I, 1945, 253–331, 694–722; and No. V, 1949, 309–32, 471–506.

Loewenthal, L. J. A., 'The Palms of Jezebel', *Folklore*, Vol. 83, 1972, 20–40.

Machado Filho, Aires da Mata, *O Negro e o Garimpo em Minas Gerais*, Rio de Janeiro, 1964.

Mackenzie, D. A., 'Colour Symbolism', *Folklore*, Vol. XXXIII, 1922, 136–69.

Maclagan, R. C., *Evil Eye in the Western Highlands*, Menston, 1972. (First published, London, 1902.)

Maclean, Una, *Magical Medicine. A Nigerian Case-Study*, London, 1974.

Madsen, William 'The Nahua', in *Handbook of Middle American Indians*, Vol. 8, Texas, 1969, 602–37.

Magalhães, Jósa, *Medicina Folclórica*, Fortaleza, 1966.

Majasan, J. A., 'Folklore as an Instrument of Education among the Yoruba', *Folklore*, Vol. 80, 1969, 41–59.

Marquès-Rivière, J., *Amulettes, Talismans et Pantacles*, Paris, 1950.

Martius, Carlos Friedr. Phil. von, *Natureza, Doenças, Medicina e Remedios dos Indios Brasileiros*, São Paulo, 1939. (First published, Munich, 1844.)

Mauss, Marcel, *A General Theory of Magic*, London, 1972. Trans. Robert Brain. (First published in *Sociologie et Anthropologie*, 1950.)

Maynard Araújo, Alceu, 'Ex-Votos ou Promessas', *Habitat*, Vol. X, São Paulo, 1952.

——, 'Alguns Ritos Mágicos', *R.A.M.*, Vol. CLXI, 1958, 45–162.

——, *Medicina Rústica*, São Paulo, 1961.

Mead, Richard, *A Treatise Concerning the Influence of the Sun and Moon upon Human Bodies*, London, 1708.

Menezes, A. Inacio de, *Flóra da Bahia*, São Paulo, 1949.

Menezes, Jayme de Sá, *Medicina Indígena (na Bahia)*, Bahia, 1957.

Métraux, A. (1) *La Religion des Tupinamba et ses rapports avec celle des autres tribus Tupi-Guaraní*, Paris, 1928. (2) *La Civilisation matérielle des tribus Tupi-Guaraní*, Paris, 1928.

——, 'The Purí-Coroado Linguistic Family', *H.S.A.I.*, Vol. I, Washington, 1946. 523–30.

——, and Baldus, 'The Guaki', *H.S.A.I.*, Vol. I, Washington, D.C., 1946, 435–44.

Montelius, Oscar, 'The Sun-God's Axe and Thor's Hammer', *Folklore*, Vol. XXI, 1910, 60–78.

Moraes Filho, Mello, *Festas e Tradições Populares do Brasil*, Rio de Janeiro, 1946.

Murphy, R., and Murphy, Y., *Women of the Forest*, New York and London, 1974.

McGregor, Pedro, *The Moon and Two Mountains—The Myths, Ritual and Magic of Brazilian Spiritism*, London, 1966.

McKenzie, Dan, *The Infancy of Medicine*, London, 1927.

M'Clintock, L., 'Donegal Cures and Charms', *Folklore*, Vol. XXIII, 1912, 473–8.

Newman, L. F., 'Some Notes on Folk Medicine in the Eastern Counties', *Folklore*, Vol. LVI, 1945, 349–60.

Nunes, Neusa, 'Benzeduras Usadas em Tubarão', *S.C.C.F.*, 5, 1950, 43–7.

Oberg, K., *Indian Tribes of Northern Mato Grosso, Brazil*, Washington, D.C., 1953.
Oesterreich, T. K., *Possession, Demoniacal and Other Among Primitive Races in Antiquity, the Middle Ages, and Modern Times*, London, 1930.
Oliveira, Sebastião Almeida, *Folclore e Outros Temas*, n.p. (São Paulo ?), 1948.
Orico, Oswaldo, *Vocabulário de Crendices Amazonicas*, São Paulo, 1937.
OSMA, *Catálogo de Azabaches Compostelanos*, Madrid, 1916.
Ott, Carlos, *Formação e Evolução Étnica da Cidade do Salvador*, Vols. I and II, Salvador, 1955.
——, 'Os "Bailes Pastoris" da Bahia', in *Bailes Pastoris na Bahia*, Salvador, 1957, 179–272.
Pardal, Ramón, *Medicina Aborigena Americana*, Buenos Aires, 1937.
Parrinder, E. G., *West African Religion*, London, 1969. (First published, London, 1949.)
——, *African Traditional Religion*, London, 1968. (First published London, 1954.)
Paula, Jefferson Davis de, 'Benzeduras Usadas em Jaraguá do Sul', *S.C.C.F.*, No. 7, 1951, 27–9; and No. 12, 1952, 16–19.
——, 'Comentários ao Vocabulário de Consultório', *S.C.C.F.*, No. 11, 1952, 46–52.
Paz, Horácio, 'Cousas do Folclore Sul-Riograndense', *S.C.C.F.*, Nos. 20/21, 1954, 72–6.
Penna, Meira, *Dicionário Brasileiro de Plantas Medicinais*, Rio de Janeiro and São Paulo, 1946.
Pettigrew, T. J., *On Superstitions Connected with the History and Practice of Medicine and Surgery*, London, 1844.
Piazza, Walter F., 'As Verrugas no Folclore Catarinense', *S.C.C.F.*, No. 2, 1949, 17–18.
——, *Folclore de Brusque—Estudo de uma Comunidade*, n.p., 1960.
Pierson, Donald, *Cruz das Almas—A Brazilian Village*, Washington, D.C., 1951.
——, *Negroes in Brazil. A Study of Race Contact at Bahia*, Carbondale, Ill., 1967.
Pinto, Estevão, *Os Indígenas do Nordeste*, São Paulo, 1935.
Piso, Guilherme, *Historia Naturalis Brasiliae*, Amsterdam, 1648. Trans. into Portuguese by Alexandre Correia, São Paulo, 1948.
Pliny, *Natural History*, Book II, London, 1938. Trans. H. Rackham.
Puckett, Newbell Niles, *Folk Beliefs of the Southern Negro*, London, 1926.
Querino, Manuel, *Costumes Africanos no Brasil*, Rio de Janeiro, 1938.
——, *A Raça Africana e os seus Costumes*, Salvador, 1955.
Radin, P., *Indians of South America*, New York, 1942.
Ramos, Arthur, *O Negro Brasileiro*, São Paulo, 1940.
——, *As Culturas Negras no Novo Mundo*, Rio de Janeiro, 1946.
——, *O Folklore Negro do Brasil*, São Paulo, 1954. (First published, Rio de Janeiro, 1935.)
——, *O Negro na Civilização Brasileira*, São Paulo, 1956.
Redinha, José, *Etnossociologia do Nordeste de Angola*, Braga, 1966.
Reichel-Dolmatoff, G., *Amazonian Cosmos, The Sexual and Religious Symbolism of the Tukano Indians*, Chicago, 1971. (First published, Bogotá, 1968.)
Rémy, N., *Demonolatry*, London, 1930. (First published, 1595.)
Ribeiro, René, *Cultos Afrobrasileiros de Recife: Um estudo de ajustamento social*,

Boletim do Instituto Joaquim Nabuco, Recife, 1952.
——, 'Brazilian Messianic Movements', in Thrupp, S. L. (ed.), *Millenial Dreams in Action—Studies in Revolutionary Religious Movements*, New York, 1970.
Risco, Vicente, 'Apuntes sobre el Mal de Ojo en Galicia', *R.D.T.P.*, Vol. XVII, 1961, 66–92.
Rivail, Léon Hippolyte Dénisart, *Le Livre des esprits contenant les principes de la doctrine spirite*, Paris, 1857.
——, *Le Spiritisme à sa plus simple expression*, Paris, 1864.
Rodrigues, Nina, *O Animismo Fetichista dos Negros Brasileiros*, Rio de Janeiro, 1935. (First published, Bahia, 1900.)
Rodrigues, Pedro Padre, 'Vida do Padre José de Anchieta', *Annaes da Bibliotheca Nacional do Rio de Janeiro*, Vol. XXIX, 1907.
Rodríguez López, J., *Supersticiones de Galicia y preocupaciones vulgares*, Lugo, 1974. (First published, 1895.)
Rolleston, J. D., 'The Folklore of Children's Diseases', *Folklore*, Vol. LIV, 1943, 287–307.
Romero, S., *Folclore Brasileiro*, Vols. 1–3, Rio de Janeiro, 1954.
Rosenberg, Tobias, *Curiosos Aspectos de la Terapéutica Calchaquí*, Tucumina, 1939.
Rozeira, Arnaldo de Mariz, 'Santo Antonio num Responso Popular', *A.C.I.E.*, 1963, 549–60.
Safford, W. E., 'Narcotic Plants and Stimulants of the Ancient Americans', *Annual Report of the Board of Regents of the Smithsonian Institution*, 1916, Washington, D.C., 1917.
St Clair, David, *Drum and Candle*, New York, 1971.
São Paulo, Fernando, *Linguagem Médica Popular no Brasil*, Vols. I–II, São Paulo, 1970. (First published, São Paulo, 1943.)
Schrire, T., *Hebrew Amulets. Their Decipherment and Interpretation*, London, 1966.
Seligmann, Kurt, *The History of Magic*, New York, 1948.
Sidney Hartland, E., 'Cleft Ashes for Infantile Hernia', *Folklore*, Vol. VII, 1896, 303–6.
Silva, Clodomir, *Minha Gente* (*Costumes de Sergipe*), Rio de Janeiro, 1926.
Simpson, G. E., 'The Shango Cult in Nigeria and Trinidad', *A.A.*, Vol. 64, No. 6, 1962, 1204–19.
Smith, E. W., *African Ideas of God*, London, 1966. (First published, London, 1950).
Southey, Robert, *History of Brazil*, Vols. I–III, London, 1810.
Speck, F. G., 'Catawba Herbals and Curative Practices', *J.A.F.*, LVII, No. 223, 1944, 37–50.
Spence, Lewis, *An Encyclopaedia of Occultism*, London, 1920.
Stade, Hans, of Hesse, 'The Captivity of Hans Stade of Hesse in A.D. 1547–1555 among the wild tribes of Eastern Brazil', annotated by Richard F. Burton, trans. A. Tootal, *The Hakluyt Society*, Vol. 51, 1874.
Summers, M., *Witchcraft and Black Magic*, Essex, 1945.
Taboada, Jesus, 'La Medicina Popular en el Valle de Monterrey (Orense)', *R.D.T.P.*, Vol. III, 1947, 31–57.

——, 'Folklore Astronómico y Meteorológico de la Comarca de Monterrey', *R.D.T.P.*, Vol. V, 1949, 110–37.
——, 'La Noche de San Juan en Galicia', *R.D.T.P.*, 1952, 600–32.
——, 'Folklore de Verín', *R.D.T.P.*, Vol. XV, 1959, 292–312.
Talbot, Percy Amaury, *The Peoples of Southern Nigeria*, Vols. 1–4, London, 1926.
Tavares, O., *Bahia: Imagens da Terra e do Povo*, Rio de Janeiro, n.d.
Teixeira, Fausto, *Medicina Popular Mineira*, Rio de Janeiro, 1954.
Teixeira, José A., *Folklore Goiano*, São Paulo, 1941.
Thomas, Keith, *Religion and the Decline of Magic*, London, 1971.
Thorndike, Lynn, *A History of Magic and Experimental Science*, Vols. I and II, New York, 1947. (First published, New York, 1923.)
True, Rodney H., 'Folk Materia Medica', *J.A.F.*, XIV, 1901, 105–14.
Valle, Cabral, 'Canções Populares da Bahia', *Gazeta Literaria*, Anno 1, No. 11, Rio de Janeiro, March 1884, 217–23.
Valle, Carlos, 'Supertições do Povo (Medicina Mágica)', *A.C.I.E.*, 1963, 595–620.
Vasconcellos, J. Leite de, *Tradições Populares de Portugal*, Porto, 1882.
——, *Sur les Amulettes Portugaises*, Lisbon, 1892.
——, *Ensaios Etnográficos*, Vols. I–III, Lisbon, 1906.
——, *A Figa*, Porto, 1925.
——, *Romanceiro Português*, Vol. I, Coimbra, 1958; Vol. II, Coimbra, 1960.
Verger, Pierre, *Notes sur le Culte des Oriṣa et Vodun à Bahia, la Baie de tous les saints, au Brésil et à l'ancienne Côte des Esclaves en Afrique*, Mémoires de l'Institut Français d'Afrique Noire, No. 51, Dakar, 1957.
Vianna Filho, Luiz, *O Negro na Bahia*, Rio de Janeiro, 1946.
Vieira Filho, Domingos, *S.C.C.F.*, Ano V, December 1953–June 1954, No. 17/19, 41–7.
Vogel, Virgil J., *American Indian Medicine*, New York, 1970.
Wagley, Charles, *Race and Class in Rural Brazil*, UNESCO, Holland, 1963. (First published, 1952.)
Waite, Arthur Edward, *The Book of Ceremonial Magic*, London, 1911.
Wallis, Budge, E. A., *Syrian Anatomy, Pathology and Therapeutics*, Vols. I and II, Oxford, 1913.
——, *The Divine Origin of the Craft of the Herbalist*, London, 1928.
——, *Amulets and Superstitions*, Oxford, 1930.
Welsford, E., *The Fool*, London, 1968. (First published, 1935.)
Wetherell, James, *Stray Notes from Bahia*, Liverpool, 1860.
Williams, Paul V. A., 'Some recent developments in an Afro-Brazilian Religion', *Anthropos*, Vol. 74, 1979, 47–54.
——, 'Exú: the master and the slave in Afro-Brazilian religion', Williams, Paul V. A., *The Fool and the Trickster: Studies in honour of Enid Welsford*, Cambridge, 1979.
Wilson, Bryan, *Magic and the Millennium*, St Albans, 1975. (First published, 1973.)
Wingate, J. S., 'The Scroll of Cyprian: an Armenian Family Amulet', *Folklore*, Vol. XLI, 1930, 169–87.

INDEX

Individual herbs, saints, and *orixás* are not listed every time they appear in the text but only when they are considered to be of particular importance or significance.

Saints' names are generally given in the form in which they first appear in the text.